ESC
Computer Pain:

Seven Commandments
of Ergonomics

Irene Chappell, B.Sc. O.T.
Occupational Therapist

ISBN: 978-0-9919363-0-4

CONTENTS

ACKNOWLEDGEMENTS

Thank you to:

Jim Chappell for his continued support, encouragement and last-minute availability to be photographed. Sophie Chappell for inspiring me daily with her unwavering work ethic. Ruth Hobbs for her patience and persistence in formatting and her unfailing willingness to problem solve. Bronwen Jorel for her "eagle eye", sense of humour and editing prowess. Lynn Laporte and her daughter Jordana for creating the clever book title. Mary Mohl, my sister, for always being there through thick and thin. Charlene Wharton for her strong and capable leadership that lessened my work load and so facilitated the writing of this book. Larry Wayland for his talents with solving formatting issues with the pictures. My two book clubs for their enthusiasm for a new book.

DEDICATION

In memory of my mother and father, who worked tirelessly all their lives to provide for their family.

My goal in creating the Seven Commandments of Ergonomics is to prevent work-related pain and to bring relief to those who work with such pain, so that they can provide for their family as my parents provided for theirs.

INTRODUCTION

Seven Commandments
of Ergonomics

A Dangerous Occupation:

C hances are that you're reading this because you've suffered a computer-related injury. If so, you're not alone. Computer-related injury is the fastest growing and least controlled work-related injury in present-day history. Considering at least 50% of the world's population works in some form of office[i] and computer use is advancing with lightning speed, computer-related injury is set for pandemic proportions.

When the average person thinks about dangerous occupations, they don't visualize a computer user. They think about people like construction workers, truck drivers, fire fighters, and the police – people who face obvious risks in their day-to-day work and who are likely to suddenly experience an obvious injury as a result. In comparison to those obviously risky professions, we computer users are a dull and unglamorous bunch. But that doesn't mean we don't get injured in the line of duty. In fact, work-related soft tissue injuries are the most frequent type of lost-time injury and the largest source of lost-time worker compensation costs in Canada. Over the last 10 years, 42% of all accepted WorkSafe claims in British Columbia were related to overexertion injuries: in other words, soft tissue injury.

On a global basis, Great Britain reports that 44% of all claims in 2010/2011 were related to soft tissue injuries.[ii] The European Agency for Safety and Health indicates that 40% of all reported injuries were musculoskeletal disorders.[iii] The United States Bureau of Labor Statistics (2009) indicates that more than a third of private-industry workers who had to take time off work did so as a result of injuries that today's office workers are likely to suffer.[iv]

What makes the modern office setting so dangerous? In a word, computers. And that's where I come in. As an occupational therapist specializing in helping injured workers return to work over the past 25+ years, I've identified the dangers inherent with computer use. And having identified them, I've developed a system that involves only seven steps to make computer use less dangerous. Do I save lives? Not in the same way that, say, a surgeon does. But I do save lives from being destroyed by the pain of computer-related injuries; I do save lives from the financial stresses that can ensue when someone is unable to work as a result of those injuries; and if you read this book and put my Seven Commandments of Ergonomics into practice, one of the lives I save in those ways could be yours.

A Silent Epidemic:

Computer users don't realize how dangerous their jobs are! We think that office work is pretty safe, but I can't count the people I've met over the last 25+ years who are unable to work because of a computer-related injury – think about the number of computer users you've seen wearing wrist braces at work. So what, exactly, is the danger?

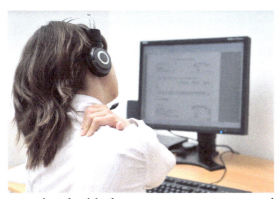

The answer is: nothing obvious; just ordinary, innocent little movements. But they're everyday little movements that are repeated over and over again, each and every working day, for years. The forces associated with these movements are so minute that the signs of danger begin innocently, almost imperceptibly. At first, you have a vague sense of discomfort and may notice one part of your body in comparison to the rest. The discomfort is easy to ignore at this stage. Little by little, however, this body part begins to demand increasing amounts of your attention, signaling greater danger; and finally the discomfort turns into pain that's impossible to ignore. It's this pain that causes days off work, sometimes months off work. While it may sound like fun to have time off work, believe me, it's no fun if you have pain that doesn't go away and prevents you from doing anything; and it's even less fun if lost earnings mean that financial stress is added to the mix.

The dangers of computer use were first identified in the 1990s, as a growing number of computer users were diagnosed with computer-related injuries and found themselves unable to work. This was described in the medical literature as a silent epidemic: "silent" because the injuries started slowly and took a long time to surface, "silent" because insurance agencies didn't want to bring attention to them, "silent" because the injuries were labeled with different terms and no one understood they were one and the same injury. Terms like carpal tunnel syndrome, repetitive strain injury, overuse injury, or cumulative trauma began to be identified in the 1980s in the medical literature, but these were all different terms for the same phenomenon. It took 10 years for the medical profession to determine that the numerous different labels given to various computer-related injuries were all the same phenomenon caused by the same things.

The "silent epidemic" of the 1990s was a result of computer use, which basically began in the 1980s. The computers of the 1960s and early 1970s had been huge, hideously expensive, and so hot (due to the large number of heat-generating semiconductors they utilized) that they were kept in a separate, cooled room. By the 1980s, however, computers were smaller, cheaper, and cooler in both senses of the word. They became more user-friendly and more affordable. Computers were quickly found to be invaluable for word processing, and companies began to replace the typewriter with the computer. Typically the typewriter table became the home for the new computer. By the 1990s, there was a 10-year history of computer use; and then came the internet, which resulted in a faster changeover, with more companies switching from the typewriter to the computer.

The introduction of the internet not only opened the doors to what we now call the information age, it also paved the way for the silent epidemic to become a pandemic. Combine the internet with the various computer devices we now have, such as laptops, phones, iPads, tablets, etc., and you realize that it's not just office workers who are experiencing computer-related injuries. Computers are everywhere. They're in offices, in schools, in retirement homes. They're part of our work life and our social life. Computers are part of hand-held mobile devices, which means that we now carry computers in our purses or in our pockets, and we take our computers everywhere we go; we use them to listen to music, send messages and receive them, record videos and watch them, take pictures and share them, and of course we play computer-related games. But just as computer use has multiplied, so has the number of computer-related injuries, and such injuries are no longer limited to one occupation (i.e., office workers) or one age group. It's true that younger people have *more* claims, because there are more young people using computers; but older people use computers too, and when they're injured, older people have *longer* claims because they don't heal as quickly.

Computer-related injuries are affecting workers, students, families, work places, the medical system and society in general. In as little as three years, a computer user can develop shoulder strain, thumb disease, flexor tendinitis, lateral epicondylitis or carpal tunnel syndrome as a result of performing the ordinary movements related to keyboarding and answering the telephone.[v][vi] Just using a mouse for more than 20 hours a week can increase your exposure to injury.[vii] Using a mobile device for three to five hours a day can cause shoulder, neck and thumb pain.[viii] Even students who use email for just 30 minutes a day on a mobile device increase their chances of experiencing shoulder pain.[ix]

Computer-related injuries are a reality. They make us non-productive. They overtax the medical system and disrupt society when they prevent us from earning a wage and supporting ourselves or our family, or when they preclude learning in school or enjoying leisure activities. Computer injury is indeed a pandemic, and an expensive one. Some people are paying in terms of pain, others in terms of lost earnings and even lost careers.

How do you ESC computer-related injuries?

Ergonomic programming and ergonomic equipment were recognized in the 1990s as important in controlling computer-related injuries, and they continue to be important today, with the most benefit occurring if posture is improved and workers incorporate breaks into the monotony of their work.[x] So why are computer-related injuries still occurring in the 2010s, and why are so many people (not just office workers) suffering?

Basically, ergonomics is not easily understood. Some think, oh, the furniture makers or equipment makers must have ergonomics already figured out and already built into the equipment I'm using. For the most part this is true, but the majority of people I work with have never adjusted the equipment they've been given, to make it fit their individual body and work habits. Some feel they're too busy to really think about ergonomics and implement it into their computer use. Others don't believe injuries can really happen to them. Some computer users try to implement ergonomic changes but discover that the information they've found isn't easy to implement. There's plenty of information out there, but it's scattered throughout the internet world.

That's why I developed the Seven Commandments of Ergonomics in the first place. I intend to deliver, in one neat package, the ergonomic information you need to work injury-free. I've developed a method you can systematically use to avoid computer-related injuries. Based on my experience over 25+ years, these are seven things that no one tells you when you start to use a computer. These seven rules will help you to avoid injury or (if it's too late for avoidance) help to decrease the pain you're experiencing from using the computer. To be fully effective, they must be implemented one at a time, starting with Commandment #1. How will these Seven Commandments prevent computer-related injury? Well, let's talk for a minute about the causes of such injuries.

The truth behind the silent epidemic:

Most of us these days have heard of terms like carpal tunnel syndrome, repetitive strain injury, overuse injury, or overexertion injury, all of which were identified and listed in the medical literature in the 1980s. What you may not have known before you read this material is that these are all different terms for the same phenomenon: injuries that are related to repetition and force. All these terms did eventually get lumped together under one heading: "musculoskeletal injury", or MSI for short. In the present-day medical literature, MSI refers to an injury or disorder of the soft tissues of the body. This includes your muscles, tendons, ligaments, joints, nerves, blood vessels or related soft tissues.

What you may not have known before reading this is that *everything* in your body is soft tissue except for the skeleton (which, as you know, consists of bone). The average skeleton weighs only 12 pounds, so if you weigh 150 pounds, this means that 138 pounds of your body – that's 92%! - is made up of soft tissue. And since MSI is damage to the soft tissue, this means that if you use a computer, a *huge* majority of your body is at risk for injury. Remember, it's performing ordinary, everyday little movements that makes computer use dangerous and causes MSI. And while we might well get wiser as we get older, I also have to point out that the older you get, the more prone you are to MSI, because you've already been doing these ordinary movements longer than your younger colleagues have. MSI was first identified and only became an epidemic <u>after</u> 10 years of computer use. MSI is a silent phenomenon that occurs as we age and gain more experience, because the longer we use the computer, the more dangerous it becomes. Sometimes life just doesn't seem fair, does it?

We tend to think about computer-related injuries as occurring only in the fingers, hands, and wrists, because those are the body parts that are most obviously associated with repetitive movement like keyboarding or using the mouse. We use the small muscles of our body to move our fingers and wrists when we work on our computer. But it's not keyboarding or mousing alone that causes MSI. Other body parts are affected not just by what they're doing but by what they're *not* doing. In the case of computer users, while the fingers are dancing over the keyboard, the rest of the body is doing nothing. For hours on end, every working day, the back, shoulders and head are held in one position (and probably an anatomically incorrect position, at that) while the hands do all the work. The result? MSI not just in the fingers, hands, and wrists, but also in the neck, shoulders, arms, and back. Pain is caused by *some* ordinary movements being performed too *many* times and *other* ordinary movements being performed too *few* times, without consideration of posture.

It would have been very hard to predict these computer-related injuries before the information age because it was very natural to assume that computers were just glorified typewriters – in fact, they were arguably typewriters that should cause *less* stress on the body because they required less force to depress the keys. You never saw typists wearing wrist braces to work or heard of them reporting typing-related injuries. Why not?

The answer is so simple it may surprise you, especially if you've never typed on a manual typewriter. Stop and think for a moment about how a typewriter used to work. Near the end of each typed line, a warning bell would ping and the typist would take her hand off the keys for long enough to pull the carriage return lever, thus sending the typewriter carriage back to its start position on the left. Naturally she also stopped typing as she did this. The typist would also take her hands off the keys when she paused to correct any errors she might make. (Hands up, all those who remember Liquid Paper or Tipp-Ex.) And when she finished typing a page, the typist had to take her hands off the keys yet again, in order to take out her typed page and put in a fresh sheet of paper. These momentary extraneous activities served a valuable function. Each time the typist was forced to take her hands off the keys, she was actually taking a tiny rest from typing, and as you can see, there were many of these natural micro-breaks in her working day. Brief though they were, each micro-break gave the typist's body a chance for recovery from the repetitive movements required for typing. The action performed during each micro-break caused a change in the typist's posture, and these changes in posture gave the body a chance for physiological recovery.

The introduction of computers put an end to all that. Computers eliminated the need to stop typing. With computers, people could type for as long as they wanted to, without having to pause. That's one of the things that make computer use dangerous: the elimination of the micro-break and, with it, the chance for physiological recovery.

The majority of the people I see with computer-related pain believe that they have no time to take a break; they feel that they have far too much work to do and that a break would slow them down. They're wrong, of course – in fact, they're painfully wrong – because in the end, it's the failure to take numerous tiny breaks that forces them to take one long, extended break, often without pay.

Let's assume that you can type 60 words a minute, based on five letters comprising a word. At this speed, which is by no means a fast one in typing terms (I know people who can type at over 100 words a minute), you'll move your fingers 300 times in a minute. Multiply that by 60 and you realize you're moving your fingers 18,000 times in an hour. Think 18,000 is a lot? Multiply it by the eight hours of an average workday. Yep, you're moving those fingers 144,000 times a day. Can you do *anything* 144,000 times a day and not have it affect you in some way? Now multiply by five and you realize that you're performing those same little movements 720,000 times a week. And that's not counting any emails you may send or documents you may create during your leisure time.

Are you starting to recognize the dangers of using a computer? Computer-related injuries are caused by the overuse of the body's smaller muscle groups and the underuse of its larger ones. But the catch is that at the time, we don't notice the overuse, let alone the underuse. We don't notice it because computer-related pain (and eventual injury) is caused by nothing more alarming than ordinary repetitive movements that use the small muscles in your body, combined with a lack of movement in the large muscle groups of your body. Add poor posture and the requirement to exert force (the more forces, the greater the danger), and you have a recipe for MSI that exponentially increases with age.

Why Ergonomics?

Before we get into why ergonomics works, let's first clarify what ergonomics actually is. Simply put, ergonomics is the study of people at work. Ergonomics, then, looks at the fit of tools and equipment in relation to the size and shape of the user, and strives to match these so as to both promote comfort and increase productivity at work. It became popular in the 1990s during the "silent epidemic" and was identified as one of the most effective methods of intervention for computer-related pain.

Whether you recognize it or not, ergonomics is part of your daily life. The whole idea behind ergonomics is to make things physically easier and more comfortable. Examples of ergonomics are everywhere. Large-grip cooking utensils, for instance, allow you to use less force when gripping. A shovel or rake with a long handle causes you to bend your back less and thus protects your spine. The option to adjust the seat height or low-back support in your car is an example of ergonomics. The only trouble with ergonomics is that people aren't taught to use ergonomic tools or principles.

Like most things in life, ergonomics can be used in either a positive way or a negative one. Recently, for example, when I went into a coffee shop with a friend, the first thing to catch my eye was two large chairs in front of the fireplace, looking comfortable and inviting. By the time I purchased my coffee, however, the comfy chairs were taken, and there were only wooden chairs remaining. (I'm sure you have days like that, too.)

The wooden chairs looked attractive in a rather contemporary way: they were high and had neither foot rest nor back support. As soon as I sat down, however, I realized that my feet were dangling in mid-air and I couldn't lean back. In fact, I quickly became so uncomfortable that I decided to leave the coffee shop and walk with my coffee instead. My chair was immediately taken by another customer, but I doubt that they stayed long either. Professionally speaking, my first thought was that the owners of the coffee shop needed some education on ergonomics, but then I realized I was wrong. These owners knew *exactly* what they were doing, ergonomically speaking. They had used ergonomics to their advantage by offering patrons a vision of two comfortable chairs in which they could relax while they sipped their coffee at leisure. And they had used ergonomics negatively by making sure that the rest of the chairs were of the uncomfortable wooden variety that would make people choose to leave quickly. This guaranteed a greater through-flow of customers and more sales for the coffee shop. Quite clever, really.

Employers don't intentionally use ergonomics to cause computer-related pain in their employees. After all, they don't want lost days of work or decreased productivity. Yet some employers fear ergonomics, thinking it will be expensive to implement. As these pages will show, it needn't be.

Ergonomics in the workplace is intended to *maximize productivity*, which is best achieved by ensuring that the worker is physically comfortable. That seems fairly obvious, and yet it's interesting to me how little thought goes into the purchase of office equipment. The work station may be initially set up by a person who knows relatively little about ergonomics and who has been told to spend as little as possible. This problem may then be compounded when a new worker comes into the office environment. Employees tend to accept what they're given, especially in tough economic times. The new employee sits down at their work station, often not really understanding why the equipment is arranged and adjusted the way it is, but taking for granted that it's that way for a reason nonetheless. This often results in the new employee immediately forming some bad habits. In an effort to see around the glare on their screen, for example, they may crane their neck or contort their body into various awkward postures. Down the road, such habits can lead to work-related MSIs.

In my experience, good ergonomics is easily added to any workplace and generally involves repositioning of equipment already owned by the employer but not always adjusted to the size and shape of the computer user. Ergonomics implemented correctly in the workplace helps to meet the bottom line as well as quickly boosting the wellbeing of the employee. This works to retain the employee and allows experienced workers to keep working, injury-free.

I want to teach you to use ergonomics to your advantage, to make the best use of the equipment you have, to control the dangers of using a computer and ultimately to avoid computer injury. Most of the people I see have heard of ergonomics; most of them have ergonomic equipment; but they've never been taught how to use ergonomics to their advantage. Ergonomics sounds like mumbo-jumbo to them. They don't understand how to use ergonomic principles to suit their particular body build and their job tasks. And that's what my Seven Commandments of Ergonomics are designed to teach you. I want to keep you working, pain-free, for as long as you want to work. Why? Because I believe that being able to work is important, and I believe that people want to work – work gives a sense of identity, of purpose, and it allows a person to support a family and contribute to society. If I can be a small part of keeping you working happily and healthily, all the information I've gathered over the last 25+ years will have been put to good use.

Why Seven Commandments of Ergonomics?

Keeping yourself injury-free involves understanding the clues your body is giving you and then responding to those clues. It means learning to use ergonomics to your advantage, and I'm here to show you how to do this in seven straightforward steps. I call these steps commandments because they're far more important than mere rules: they're critical in preventing pain and injury when you work with a computer. Following these Seven Commandments of Ergonomics in sequence will allow you to adjust your work station to fit *you*; it will give you power over your work; and it will allow you to keep working in a healthy way. As you understand and apply these Seven Commandments, you'll get rid of the pain you now experience as a result of computer use, and what's more, you'll prevent that MSI pain from returning in the future.

What makes me so sure I can help with *your* problems? Well, when I get called in to help someone who's having computer-related pain, the ergonomic problems I find are always the same, so it's a pretty safe bet that you have the same ergonomic problems too. In every case, I find that the same seven things need to be adjusted so that the computer station fits the worker. Not only do the same seven things always need to be adjusted, but they always need to be adjusted in the same order. The seated posture is where the problems all stem from. When I use one or more of these seven commandments to match the computer user's individual body shape and size to the equipment they're using, that person has less pain when working. Following the Seven Commandments of Ergonomics, I haven't had a failure yet! In some cases, pain decreases instantly; in other cases, it may take a few days; but in every case, sooner or later benefit is achieved.

Once you learn to recognize the clues your body is giving you, you can respond to the clues by using the Seven Commandments of Ergonomics. If you have MSI pain related to computer use, following the seven commandments will control the pain. The commandments will provide you with a system to follow in order to fit your tools and equipment to your own unique body build and your own computer work station. Each commandment in turn considers your size, your height, your body build and your work method. With each commandment you implement, your body is better positioned to perform your work tasks, making you better able to cope with the stresses of repetition and force that are inherent in the ordinary movements you perform daily. By following the Seven Commandments of Ergonomics, you'll be able to adjust your chair and position your keyboard, mouse, monitor, telephone, etc., so that the soft tissues of your body can better cope with the demands of the ordinary movements of your work.

With the use of each commandment, your body will be moved closer to the correct anatomical posture. You may be surprised to learn that it's posture that's the common denominator in all seven commandments. It's working in your correct posture that's the key to fighting the biomechanical and physiological stresses that cause computer injury. The trick, of course, is first to know what correct posture is, and second to know how to set up your work station so that correct posture is your default position when you're working.

Escape Computer Pain with the Seven Commandments of Ergonomics:

I formulated the Seven Commandments of Ergonomics over the last 25 years, after performing many, many ergonomic assessments dealing with many, many computer-related problems. We'll be covering these commandments in the upcoming chapters, each of which will start with the case history of an actual ergonomic assessment I performed. (Names and identifying details have, of course, been altered for privacy reasons.) There will be step-by-step instructions on how to carry out each commandment, including pictures to help guide your intervention. Where applicable, I'll throw in a brief anatomy lesson to illustrate the anatomical and biomechanical reasons behind the commandment. At the end of the seven chapters explaining each commandment, you'll find a chapter with a checklist and at-a-glance instructions that you can use to adjust your own work station. If you don't change your work station in the order given, starting with the first commandment, you'll find yourself rearranging your work space a multiple number of times, and definitely more than seven. Believe me, I've been there. Please do work through the chapters in order, because I've found from experience that the steps work best if performed in the sequence outlined below.

This book will show you how to use the power of ergonomics to your advantage. But don't just read it – you need to apply it as well. If you diligently carry out the Seven Commandments of Ergonomics, you'll have performed an ergonomic consultation and intervention on your own work station. And that's one of my goals – to teach people how to perform their own ergonomic assessment so that they can work in a way that minimizes their risk of injury. If only 1% of office workers use these seven steps, millions of dollars and dreams will be saved. My number one goal is to assist you to work comfortably and injury-free for as long as you want to work. Work smarter so you can play harder! Change the way you use your computer and you can change your financial future.

Chapter One

Commandment One

Secure the Spine

Case History:

The Problem:

When Sophie Child, a copyright lawyer in her early 30s, returned to the office from maternity leave, she expected that the most painful thing about going back to work would be missing her sweet baby girl. As it turned out, however, the most painful thing was her upper back. And within the first three days of working, the pain had intensified to such a level that she couldn't work full-time.

Sophie hadn't been aware of any warning signs, and she was totally unprepared for this turn of events. Her pregnancy had been uneventful and the birth straightforward. While on maternity leave during the first few months of her new baby's life, Sophie had had no difficulty lifting, carrying or cradling her newborn. She'd been able to perform all the usual housework; she'd done some gardening; she'd even played squash twice a week. None of these activities had caused any symptoms. Yet now, in an office environment that made few demands on her body, Sophie had apparently done something to her back that had caused so much damage she couldn't do the things she'd done while on maternity leave. She couldn't do household or gardening chores, she couldn't play squash, and worst of all, she couldn't hold her new baby for lengthy periods of time.

Since Sophie was right-handed and the pain was located in the right upper back area, she suspected it was related to her work station. Deciding that her chair was the most likely culprit, she tracked down chairs in the office that weren't being used and wheeled them to her work station. But despite trying three different types, she was still in pain.

Sophie was used to making quick decisions, so when she found that she couldn't solve the problem herself, she immediately looked for someone who *could* solve it. That's when I was asked to perform an ergonomic assessment. The Director of Human

Resources had attended a conference where I made a presentation on the Seven Commandments of Ergonomics, and she telephoned me to set up an appointment.

As you'll recall (I hope!) from the previous chapter, I consider posture to be absolutely the most important aspect in preventing and/or treating musculoskeletal injuries, so you won't be surprised to learn that when I do an ergonomic assessment of a client's computer work space, I always start by looking at their posture. My second priority is to have the client identify their most frequent job task, so that I can determine the effects of the repetitive task, the forces used in the repetitive task and how posture affects both the repetitive task and the force required.

Sophie identified her most repetitive task to be working on the computer from hard copy. As a copyright lawyer, she was continually referencing large books, multiple files, or binders and then using the keyboard to enter the information onto the computer's hard drive. While doing so, she habitually slouched in her chair, sitting with a rounded back, with the result that her trunk and shoulders were curved toward her belly. I should point out that Sophie didn't sit this way because she was lazy or slobbish. In fact, the majority of office workers tend to sit this way when they work, so there's a good chance that you do too. It's a habit that usually arises – and in Sophie's case, certainly did arise – because the worker's chair fails in one very important respect: it doesn't *secure the spine*. In other words, it promotes slouching. Her spine wasn't supported in the correct anatomical posture. Her tools and equipment weren't positioned to encourage an erect posture. Her books and binders were on a variety of different surfaces, and she had to twist her back while reading the materials and typing on the keyboard.

Naturally enough, when sitting in the slouched position I've just described, Sophie inadvertently bent her neck more than necessary in order to look down at the desktop so that she could read whatever document she happened to be working from. The forces of gravity pushed down on Sophie's neck and upper back muscles, and keeping an upright posture against the forces of gravity resulted in extra work for those muscles. Continually fighting the effects of gravity to maintain her head and back in a semi-erect posture was costing her body a good deal of energy and resulting in pain.

The Solution:

S ophie was intuitively on the right track in suspecting that her chair was causing her back pain. As simple as it sounds, the major problem was that the chair didn't support her low back curve properly – it didn't secure her spine. Because the chair didn't fit into her low back curve, it encouraged the curve to flatten against the chair and caused her shoulders to round and her head to bend forward. Because Sophie spent a long period of the day looking down onto her desk to read her hard copy, this encouraged her to slouch further. The longer the day, the more she slouched; her head posture became more bent, which made her low back posture even worse. Gravity pushed harder and harder against her neck and upper back. Later in this chapter, I'll explain how to make sure your chair *does* secure your spine, so that you can avoid the problems Sophie had. Her chair didn't support her spine in an anatomically correct posture, and the problem wasn't helped by the fact that her tools and equipment weren't positioned to encourage an anatomically correct posture either. I'll explain how to avoid that mistake, too, a little later in the book.

The first thing I did was adjust the chair Sophie was using to make it fit her unique body build. The good news was that her chair had a lumbar back support, but the bad news was that it was positioned too low to give support where she needed it most. I raised the low back support so that it fit into her lumbar spine. This change encouraged her to sit up straight, which in turn secured her spine in an anatomically correct posture.

Secondly, I gave her a dedicated reading area directly under her computer monitor. Sophie had been bending her neck too far forward when looking down onto her desktop to read her hard copy, and this had put a lot of strain on the muscles of her neck and upper back. She was also twisting her neck, which added to the strain. I don't suppose you've stopped to consider what the weight of the average human head is, so you might be surprised to learn that it weighs between 8 and 10 pounds. Next time you're sitting at your desk, try propping your elbows on the desktop while you hold a 10-pound bag of potatoes balanced on your open hands, and you'll get some idea of how much effort your neck and upper back muscles have to put into supporting your head.

To give Sophie's muscles a break, I needed to prevent her head from bending, so I raised her reading materials onto an inclined surface. Then I raised the height of her computer monitor so that she didn't have to bend her neck when she was looking at the screen. The end result was that when she was working, Sophie only needed to move her eyes: she no longer needed to bend or twist her head, and her neck could now stay in its anatomically correct position, as could her low back. She felt different immediately. By the end of the week, Sophie was working symptom-free.

Sophie's is a success story: with my help, she got rid of her back pain by using the Seven Commandments of Ergonomics, specifically Commandment #1 – *Secure the Spine*, which altered the posture she was using at her computer work station. Once Sophie's chair had been adjusted so that it provided her with correct back support, it was easy for her spine to fall into an anatomically correct posture when she was seated. Likewise, once her equipment had been moved so that she didn't need to bend or twist her neck when reading, her neck posture naturally defaulted into anatomically correct alignment as well. With her work station properly set up, Sophie was no longer distracted by pain but was free to concentrate on her work.

First Commandment of Ergonomics
Secure the Spine:

S ophie's case example illustrates the importance of securing the spine by sitting up straight in an anatomically correct posture. I'd like to give you a short anatomy lesson to help you understand *why* the position of the spine is so crucial, but don't worry, I've purposely kept it simple for ease of reference. Those of you who hated anatomy lessons in school and want to go straight to the part that deals with how to apply the rule, rather than why it works, may want to skip ahead to "How do you Secure the Spine when sitting?" but I do hope you won't. I'd like you all to stick with me for the next page or two.

The First Anatomy Lesson:

T he back or *spine* consists of a series of bones called vertebrae, whose size and shape depends on which part of the back they're located in: the neck (upper back or cervical spine), the trunk (mid back or thoracic spine) or the low back (lumbar spine).

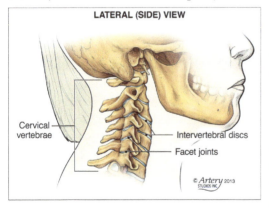

The Neck: The seven vertebrae in the neck are smaller than those in the trunk or low back. They're also flatter, with smaller bony protrusions, and they move easily. Because the head is moved by the neck, the flat construction of these vertebrae allows our head to look up at the ceiling, down at the floor, to our left and right, behind us, and at all points in between.

The Trunk: Below the neck are the 12 thoracic vertebrae which stack on one another to form our trunk (considered to be the area from your shoulders to your waist). These truncal vertebrae act to anchor our ribs and shoulder blades, and protect our internal organs. They're tall and wide, and the ribs attach directly to these vertebrae at the back and to the breastbone at the front. The thoracic vertebrae also have bony protrusions that overlap the vertebrae above and below, a configuration which acts to form a rigid cage-like structure (the rib cage) that has minimal movement. There are many important internal organs in our chest that don't like to be jostled – organs such as the heart and lungs, without which we really don't function too well – so you can see why the rib cage is such a good idea.

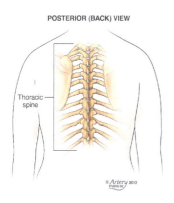

POSTERIOR (BACK) VIEW

Thoracic spine

© *Artery* 2013

The human trunk is quite heavy: it constitutes the majority of a person's total body weight. And while the average person may think the trunk is able to move in many directions, this isn't true. The trunk is rigid, and truncal movements are minimal. All movements of the trunk are provided by the low back or lumbar vertebrae. In other words, it's only when you bend or twist your low back that your trunk moves. When you understand this phenomenon, you'll understand the necessity of protecting your low back and avoiding extreme movements of the trunk.

The Low Back: The five low back vertebrae are the largest ones in our bodies, being twice the size of the vertebrae in the neck or trunk. These lumbar vertebrae are located from your waist to the upper part of your buttocks, and they make up the structure that allows your trunk to move forward, backward, and from side to side, as well as to rotate. One of the odd things about the human anatomy is that even though the lumbar vertebrae move the largest and heaviest body part, namely the trunk, there are only five of them. However, this anomaly does go a long way to explaining why most back injuries occur in the lower back.

The main objective of Ergonomic Commandment #1 – *Secure the Spine* is to align the vertebrae in their optimum position, namely, the position in which they're stacked on top of each other the way they were meant to be. And to keep your vertebrae in their anatomically correct position, you don't just align them before you start work – you have to keep them aligned while you're working. That's what I mean by *securing the spine*.

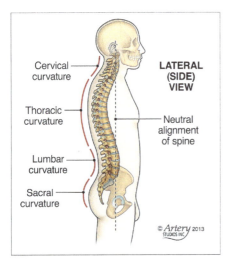

When all these vertebrae are stacked in the anatomically correct position, there's a certain shape that results: an "S" shape, with distinct curvature at the neck and low back. Look at the picture below and you'll see what I mean. The top of the S is at the neck vertebrae, then there's an outward protrusion at the level of the shoulder blade, and finally you can see the bottom of the S at the low back. You *must* maintain this curve when you're working, otherwise you won't be allowing the vertebrae to stack properly on top of one another, and you can guess where *that* will lead, can't you? Yes, back pain. (The structure of the spine is discussed in more detail in the Anatomy Lesson of Chapter Five).

In all work tasks, this S shape must be maintained in order to prevent discomfort and pain. How do you know when you're sitting in an anatomically correct position? Your ears will be positioned directly above your shoulders and your shoulders will be directly above your hips – simple as that. From an ergonomic perspective, you want to keep your ears, shoulders and hips aligned in all your work tasks.

How do you Secure the Spine when sitting?

You'll notice that I said achieving the correct sitting posture was simple. There are only five steps to complying with Commandment #1 – *Secure the Spine*, but you need to do them in the correct order. Here we go!

Step 1: Identify your low back/lumbar curve: As you'll recall, this is part of that S curve we discussed above. Put your hand behind your back, at the waist, where your belt should be if you're wearing one. Feel the curve there? That's your low back curve, alias your lumbar curve. When you're seated, this curve needs to be supported by the chair you're sitting on.

Step 2: Ensure the chair is the correct height to secure your low back curve: If your feet dangle or your knees are too high, your low back curve will be either flattened or accentuated – it won't be aligned correctly. To maintain the correct alignment of your pelvis, your knees should be bent at a 90-degree angle, and your hips should form another 90-degree angle when seated. How do you get this 90-degree angle? Stand in front of your chair. The bottom of your kneecap should be at the same height as the seat pan of the chair. If it isn't, change the height of the seat. If your kneecap is at the same height as the seat pan when you're standing, when you sit down your knee will bend to 90 degrees and so will your hips. That's the position you want: 90 in the knees and 90 in the hips.

In most cases, the lever to adjust the height of the seat pan will be on the underside of the chair, on the right-hand side. If you can't change the height of the seat, then you need a different chair.

Step 3: Support your low back curve: Your chair should, of course, have a back rest, and that back rest should in turn have a raised surface which acts as a support for the low back. Back rests are normally adjustable in an up-and-down plane, so move the back rest until its raised surface fits into your low back curve. Some back rests move forward and backward, too. Make sure the

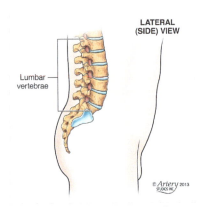

LATERAL
(SIDE) VIEW

Lumbar
vertebrae

© *Artery* 2013
STUDIOS INC.

back rest is forward enough so it supports your trunk in a posture where your ear is directly over your shoulder and your shoulder is over your hip. Once the raised surface of the back rest fits properly into your lumbar curve and the forward/backward adjustment is correct, the anatomical alignment of the three curves of the back will be naturally supported while you work: your ears will be directly over your shoulders, and your shoulders will be directly over your hips.

Step 4: Provide support to your legs: Your thighs should be supported by the seat pan of your chair in a manner that further supports your low back curve. If the seat pan of your chair is too short, even though your knees and hips started off at their correct 90-degree angles, gravity will come into play, and the weight of your legs will gradually but inevitably pull your pelvis forward. Once that happens, your lumbar curve will no longer be in anatomical alignment.

If the seat pan is the correct length for your thighs, the distance between the seat and the back of your knee will be no bigger than the size of your fist.

Some chairs have a lever that slides the seat pan forward or backward. In others, the back rest will slide forward and backward, thus increasing or diminishing distance in the seat pan.

Step 5: Correct Use of Arm Rest: Many chairs have arm rests. The correct fit of the arm rest keeps the shoulder in an anatomically neutral position. The arm rests should be positioned at a width which allows the arm to rest close to the trunk, and should be high enough so that the elbows are supported at a 90-degree bend. They should be long enough to support the length and weight of your forearm; please be aware and don't allow your wrists to hang in extreme flexion when resting on the arm rests.

Incidentally, there's no rule that says you *have* to use arm rests. In many cases, they interfere with situating yourself at the correct distance from the work surface. So if your arm rests interfere with getting as close to your work surface as you need to be, get rid of them.

Those are the five rules to make sure your chair is at the correct height and fully supports your low back curve, the length of your thighs and forearms. Did you apply the rules correctly? Let's check. After you've adjusted the low back support of your chair to your unique build, sit in your chair and you should find that your feet are flat on the floor, your knees are bent at a 90-degree angle, and your hips are also at a 90-degree angle. Put your hand behind your knee and you should find room for your fist (but no more than that) between the back of your knee and the front of the chair seat. Notice whether your low back curve is filled with the outcrop from the back rest of the chair: you shouldn't be able to put your hand between the back of the chair and your low back curve. If you have arm rests on your chair, check that they're adjusted so they barely touch your forearms when your elbows are bent at 90 degrees. So…how'd you do? If everything is where it should be, your ears are directly over your shoulders and your shoulders are directly over your hips. Congratulations! You're sitting in an anatomically correct posture. You have *Secured the Spine*!!

Summary:

Many computer users have discomfort and pain that can be directly related to the posture they assume when using their computer. Those end-of-the-day areas of discomfort you ignore eventually turn into pain, and all too often it's pain in the back or the neck. Pain is caused by the overuse of the smaller muscle groups or the underuse of the larger muscle groups, without consideration of anatomically correct posture. Your body is amazing in its construction. Your 12-pound skeleton, with hundreds of articulating parts, is shaped and sized so it can work effortlessly and efficiently when all the parts are lined up to fit together in an anatomically correct manner. All the vertebrae in the neck, trunk and lower back need to line up so that the S shape is secure. The ear must be over the shoulder and the shoulder over the hip for this to occur, regardless of whether you sit or stand. Good posture depends on securing and maintaining the spine in an anatomically correct position when you're performing your work tasks. How do you do this? Firstly, by being able to identify the anatomical landmarks of "ear over shoulder, shoulder over hip" when working. Secondly, by being able to adjust your chair to secure good posture when you're using your computer. As we've just seen, there are only five steps required to fit your chair to your unique body build. Working with a correct chair fit is the first step to **ESC Computer Pain**.

Chapter Two

Commandment Two

Beware the Chair

Case History:

The Problem:

Francine worked in human resources for a large company. She had held the same job for the past seven and a half years, and the only thing she didn't like about it was the pain.

Part of Francine's daily work involved using the computer for long periods of time while she entered information from various hard-copy sources. It wasn't until she was in her early 40s that she noticed she was becoming more aware of her right shoulder. As time went on, Francine noticed that there was a pattern to the discomfort, in that it always occurred near the end of the work day and it grew stronger as the week progressed. Every Friday, she knew she had a right shoulder, and every Monday, she was back to normal.

The discomfort slowly progressed to a nagging feeling that she experienced every day of the working week and that didn't go away with overnight rest; but at the end of each weekend, she was back to being pain-free. By the time Francine was in her mid 40s, however, she could no longer count on the shoulder pain going away with a weekend of rest. Worse than that, she couldn't get away with calling it "discomfort" or "nagging" anymore: this was pain, and she had it every single working day. It started soon after she began her daily work and intensified as the day went on. It was even waking her up at night. Francine began to worry.

She went to her chiropractor and then to a physiotherapist. Their approaches were different but the result was the same: she experienced temporary relief, but the pain returned with just a few hours of work. Francine decided to try over-the-counter medication and found that it helped to some extent: it didn't take the pain away, but at least it dulled it. But she wasn't very happy about the prospect of taking medication on a long-term basis.

I was called in to perform an ergonomic consultation when Francine began to miss multiple days off work. She's the type of worker I assess regularly: a textbook example of the experienced worker who's performed computer work for over 10 years. Performing the same physical actions over and over again for hours, weeks, months and years can take its toll. Typically the body sends hints (like the "nagging" Francine was feeling) that something isn't right, but we usually ignore the hints until we just can't ignore them any longer – until the nagging changes into pain and the pain doesn't go away.

Using the Seven Commandments of Ergonomics, I began Francine's assessment by looking at her posture while she was seated at her work space. Next, we identified the placement of her most frequently used tools. In an ergonomic consultation, it's extremely important to identify the most repetitive work tasks, in order to determine how the location of the tools and equipment used in their performance has altered the worker's anatomically correct posture. Has the placement of the tools and equipment put the individual into an awkward or static posture? If so, to what degree? How has the placement of the tools and equipment affected the forces used to complete the task?

It's probably no surprise to you to learn that Francine's most repetitive tasks were evenly split between using the keyboard and using the mouse.

Interestingly, Francine met all the criteria to satisfy Commandment #1 – *Secure the Spine*. She was sitting on a chair that she had adjusted perfectly to secure her spine. Her low back curve was supported by the lumbar support of the back of the chair. Her thighs were supported at 90 degrees, and the seat-pan length was correct when considering the length of her thighs. So Francine's problems were not caused by the chair *per se*.

Her problems were, however, most definitely related to the chair. Where Francine had gone wrong was that although she had carefully fit the chair to her body, she hadn't thought to fit the chair to her actual work space. Like most people, she wasn't aware of the importance of positioning the chair to match the tools and equipment she was using. Francine needed to *Beware the*

Chair. Not only was she was sitting at an incorrect distance from the tools she used most frequently during her work day, she was also at an incorrect height for them. She was too far away from her mouse, too high for her keyboard, and also too high for her monitor.

When she was using her mouse, Francine's right arm was stretched quite a distance away from her body, to the far right of her desk. This meant that her elbow was almost straight. What's more, her mouse was on a work surface that was at hip height. Her keyboard, on the other hand, was almost resting on her thighs. Her computer monitor was at a height that was too low. Francine had a copy holder but preferred to place her work materials flat on her desk. This meant that when she looked down at her materials, her chin was almost touching her chest. Also, when working from hard copy, she had to twist her neck to the right and look down on the desk surface. She was using awkward and unnatural postures when working. The way I've described Francine's working postures, you can identify that they sound strange and awkward, but after working in these postures over and over again for the 10 years she had been with this company (not to mention the dozen or so years of desk work before that, when she had probably used a similar position), Francine found them perfectly natural.

The Solution:

Intervening to make Francine comfortable was very easy in light of the second of the Seven Commandments of Ergonomics, *Beware the Chair*. In essence, although Francine's chair did fit her particular body type, it didn't fit the work surface. It wasn't at the correct height to the work surface, nor was it at the correct distance. To match Francine's chair to her work surface, all I had to do was match the height of the chair to the height of her most frequently used tools.

Was Francine excited about the changes? Well, not exactly. In fact, she resisted every change I suggested, even though she knew they were designed to be of benefit to her. But resistance to change is to be expected. Francine had been working in the same posture for many years, so naturally the new posture I put her in felt awkward. As with anything new, one must get used to a new *modus operandi*. I asked Francine to try the new posture for just a week, assuring her that at the end of that time, she could return to her old way of working if she wanted to. She agreed reluctantly, but she did agree. (Pain can be very persuasive.) Her keyboard, chair and monitor were all raised in height, and her mouse was moved from the desktop to the same surface as her keyboard. I wasn't surprised – but I was certainly relieved! – when after a week of working with the changed setup, Francine chose to keep it. Once the chair matched the work surface and she no longer had to reach at a diagonal to work with the mouse, she had noticed a dramatic improvement in her right shoulder pain.

Second Commandment of Ergonomics
Beware the Chair:

Francine's case example illustrates the importance of paying attention to the fit of the chair to your work space – *Beware the Chair*. If the tools and equipment you use most frequently are too far away from your body, then the forces that your body exerts to perform that task are unnecessarily amplified, and ergonomics is working to your disadvantage. Your body will be unable to handle this over the long term. The first sign of using poor ergonomics is experiencing discomfort in one particular body part. For Francine, it started with discomfort in her shoulder that began "nagging" at the end of each work day. The clue was subtle but important.

Anatomy Lesson:

Working at incorrect distances or heights from your work surface can cause discomfort, pain and injury. The wear and tear on your body structures is amplified, and you feel the effects of that strain much more quickly than you feel the effects of the same amount of work performed when the work tools are at the correct distances and/or heights. Try this little experiment. Pick up your pen and hold it in mid-air so that your arm is straight out in front of you (elbow straight, arm at shoulder height). Not much effort involved, right? Now put down the pen, put your watch on the table, pick up the pen again and time how long you can hold it in mid-air before your arm begins to become too heavy or you start to be aware of your shoulder. Most people can't hold their arm up for more than a minute. Surprising, eh? The reason it's so difficult is that even when holding something as light as a pen in mid-air, the position forces your arm to act as a long lever, thus placing you at a mechanical disadvantage. The muscles in your shoulders have to work hard to support the length and weight of your arm against gravity, and gravity starts to win the battle.

This same effect happens on a daily basis when your mouse is too far away from you, requiring your shoulder muscles to work non-stop in a static manner to support the weight of your arm. The muscles quickly lose their energy because of the lack of muscle movement which would typically replenish the blood and thus the energy supply to the muscle. (Muscle energy is discussed in detail under "The Importance of Breaks" in chapter 7). As you found if you did the experiment above, when your muscles pit themselves against the forces of gravity, eventually something has to give – and believe me, it won't be gravity. But even though we can't hope to defeat gravity completely, we can still counteract its effects on the soft tissue structures of our bodies by fitting our chair to the correct height and distance from our work surface.

Beware the Chair - How do you position your chair to your work surface?

Once you've fit the chair to your body, it's time to fit the chair to your work space. You may need to adjust your entire work station, so before you start making drastic changes, make sure your chair fits into your low back curve and your thighs are supported properly. (Please see Commandment #1 – *Secure the Spine*.) Assuming that your chair is indeed set up to secure your spine in accordance with the first commandment, here's how we go on to implement the second commandment.

Step 1. Ensure your feet are flat on the floor: If your feet dangle or your knees are too high, your low back curve won't be aligned correctly: instead, it'll be either flattened or accentuated. To maintain the correct alignment, your knees and hips should be at a 90-degree angle. How do you get that all-important angle?

Stand in front of your chair. The bottom of your kneecap should be at the same height as the seat pan of the chair. Now sit down. Your hips and knees should be at 90 degrees, and your feet should be flat on the floor.

Step 2: Identify your most frequent task, and set the correct height and distance of the chair accordingly: The correct height will have your elbow bent to 90 degrees. The correct distance is the length of your forearm.

If your most frequent task involves the keyboard: Start by sliding your chair in front of the keyboard – and as you do so, be aware of just how easily (or not!) your chair slides to your work surface, because if you have to use your feet forcefully to push the chair along, you're causing undue stresses to your spine. A low pile carpet or a plastic mat under your chair will help it slide with minimal leg thrust. Make sure the plastic mat is the same size as your rolling work surface: you don't want to slide off the edge of the mat when rolling your chair, as that causes another type of stress.

Now, place your arms beside your body so they're touching your trunk and bend your elbows so they're at a 90-degree angle. Your keyboard should be right there at your fingertips. If it isn't, then you need to change either the height of the keyboard or the height of your chair. Your goal is to be able to use the keyboard while your arms are tucked beside your trunk and your elbows are at 90 degrees: you should be able to feel your trunk with your elbows while you're typing. By keeping your arms close to your body while you work, you'll decrease the effects of gravity and diminish the muscle forces used in your shoulders, neck and low back.

Most people have their keyboard on a keyboard tray when they work, and you may even be fortunate enough to have an adjustable one, which will make it much easier for you to get a good match between the chair height, your bent elbow and the keyboard.

If, however, you have to work with your keyboard on the desk, you'll almost certainly need to raise the height of your chair in order to use the keyboard with a 90-degree elbow and make it a good match. Raising the height of your chair may mean that your feet are no longer flat on the floor, of course. You'll be tempted to think that this isn't important, but you'd be wrong, because if your feet aren't supported, your pelvis won't be supported and you'll have lost all the benefits associated with a good chair fit. So…if you have to raise the height of the chair to make it the right height for your keyboard but your feet then aren't flat on the floor, either gather up enough phone books to put under your feet to achieve that magic 90-degree angle with your knees, or better yet, buy a foot rest.

There are, of course, some rules for foot rest use. First and foremost, both feet must fit on the foot rest. Another very important factor is that it should be stable – it should not move unpredictably. Also, being able to move your ankles up and down when using the foot rest is allowable and even preferable (think muscle movement here, and fighting the effects of gravity). Foot rests come in different heights, so please be aware of your knee and hip angles: they should continue to be at 90 degrees when using a foot rest. Don't be tempted to use a foot rest that's too high; you don't *ever* want to allow your knees to be higher than your hips – not *ever*!!

If your most frequent task includes the mouse: In this case, start by sliding your chair in front of the mouse. Position the chair so that your arm is tucked close to your body, and bend your elbow so that it's at 90 degrees. The mouse should now be at your fingertips. It must be close to – and on the same work surface as – the keyboard if you're going to achieve anatomical correctness when you use it. So if your mouse isn't at your fingertips when your arm is tucked close to your trunk, you know what you need to do, don't you? Move it!!

If your most frequent task includes the monitor: The monitor should always be directly over the keyboard, so start by sliding your chair and/or repositioning the monitor so that it's directly in front of your body and also directly above the keyboard. When using the monitor, your head and neck should be straight, and your nose should be aligned with the centre of the monitor. Your chin should be parallel to the floor, and your eyebrows should be at the same level as the toolbar on your screen. (Yes, you could just raise or lower your eyebrows to get them to the right level, but no, that's not a viable long-term solution – although it would probably entertain the rest of the office.) When you meet all these criteria, you've achieved the best fit of the chair to the work station.

If your most frequent task includes a laptop: Trust me, it's impossible to position a laptop so that your arms as well as your head are in the correct position. The easiest thing to do is to plug in an external keyboard and use the laptop as a monitor. The height of the chair should, of course, position your elbows at 90 degrees when you use the external keyboard. Raise the height of the laptop so that your nose is centred, your chin is parallel to the floor, and your eyebrows are at toolbar height. You can use multiple phone books to raise the laptop, or alternatively there are many types of commercially available raisers that are mobile and very useful. Plug in that external keyboard, make sure your elbows are aligned properly at 90 degrees, and you've accomplished *Beware the Chair*!

Positioning frequent and occasional tasks: *Beware the Chair* means fitting the chair to the work surface and also to your work intensities. It means looking at your tasks and deciding which ones are performed most frequently and where each task should be performed. Use the following formula to determine what your most frequent tasks are and where they should be positioned on your work surface: If the task is performed *more* than eight times an hour, it's a frequent task and should be completed within forearm's distance from your body. If the task is performed *less* than eight times an hour, it's an occasional task and should be performed at arm's reach away from you.

Think of it this way: if you do anything more than eight times an hour, it should always be done with your elbows tucked close to your body and the equipment at your fingertips.

Although you don't use your chair when you're filing or accessing hard-copy materials, you should be aware of *securing your spine* when performing such tasks. No matter what the weight of the materials you're filing or storing, always store the most frequently used items between knuckle and shoulder height. That way, you don't have to bend your back more than 30 degrees when you access them. And when you don't bend your back, you're protecting your discs and preventing back pain. Good plan!

Summary:

One of the most commonly forgotten steps in preventing workplace injuries is one of the easiest things to fix. That step is identifying whether the most frequently used equipment and tools are situated at the right height and distance for your particular body size. The second commandment, *Beware the Chair*, is a reminder that after you fit the chair to your body, you have to fit the chair to your work surface. You do this by identifying your most frequently used tools or pieces of equipment and then adjusting the chair height and distance in relation to those items. The correct *height* will have your elbow bent to 90 degrees; the correct *distance* is the length of your forearm. Make sure you arrange your work area so that the tasks you perform more than eight times an hour are within forearm's length away and will be performed with your elbow bent at 90 degrees. Avoid any reaching postures. I know you'll be more comfortable when you can implement this step. Enjoy your work day!

Chapter Three

Commandment Three

Align the Arms

Case History:

The Problem:

S onia, an occupational therapist, was a specialist in helping injured workers return to work. She had been a work capacity specialist for more than 25 years, a job that involved assessing people who had suffered a traumatic injury and then writing a detailed report outlining whether the injured person could still fulfil each of their job duties. If the person could no longer carry out their duties, Sonia described what accommodations they would need in order to return to work. Her report writing time was extensive, sometimes taking up to 20 hours.

While it was true that Sonia used the computer for extended periods of time, she only did so on the days when she wasn't involved in performing the actual assessments, which meant that she usually worked on the computer three days a week. Sonia enjoyed her job and rarely took days off, but at the end of each computer work day, she was starting to find herself complaining of right shoulder pain. And without even realizing it, she slowly began changing her lifestyle to deal with the shoulder pain.

Sonia's first lifestyle change involved her dog. Typically, she went for long walks after work with her border collie, who loved to run. An admirer of the breed, Sonia was also involved in rescuing, fostering, and training border collies, which meant that it wasn't unusual for her to walk two or three relatively untrained dogs at once. While her own border collie was well trained and could safely be walked off leash, handling the leashes of the other dogs caused jerky movements to her right arm that aggravated her shoulder. This was particularly troublesome after a computer work day, and Sonia began to shorten her walks on those days in an effort to avoid the pain. In the end, sadly and reluctantly, she gave up fostering rescued dogs altogether, simply because of the repeated aggravation to her shoulder.

Her second lifestyle change involved gardening. Sonia had a large yard with both a flower garden and a vegetable garden, and she found them very rewarding. It was satisfying to her to plant things and watch them grow, she deeply appreciated the colour and scent of her flowers, and the intense flavor of her fresh-picked vegetables made her evening meal more enjoyable. But as her shoulder pain increased, her pleasure in gardening decreased, until one year, she didn't plant anything at all.

Sonia finally called on my services when her shoulder pain was constant despite the fact that she had given up all potentially aggravating activities except work. She had now reached the point where she was starting to limit the movements in her arm, in an effort to reduce the pain. When I interviewed her during the ergonomic assessment, she mentioned that she had injured her right shoulder 10 years earlier and had gone on to develop "frozen shoulder" or, in medical terms, adhesive capsulitis. As you may know, frozen shoulder is a condition that causes stiffness of the soft tissues of the shoulder, which in turn causes the movements of the shoulder to be painful. In Sonia's case, movement of the shoulder had become virtually impossible. However, she had diligently completed many months of physiotherapy, and after two years of rehabilitation, she had regained full movement in her right shoulder. I could hear the note of pride in her voice when she told me that her frozen shoulder symptoms had been resolved for years.

While the physiotherapy had undoubtedly helped, Sonia had also been fortunate. The symptoms of frozen shoulder do resolve, but generally this requires a lengthy period of time, and it's not uncommon for the pain and the lack of movement to last for two years. Doctors aren't sure why frozen shoulder happens to some people and not to others, but the condition tends to occur mostly in women over the age of 40.

Despite her recovery from frozen shoulder, there was no doubt that Sonia was worried about the fact that she was once again experiencing shoulder pain on the days she used a computer at work, and she was deeply concerned that she was starting to lose movement in her shoulder. Her experience was by no means unusual. I find it's typical that when an individual has injured themselves when they were younger, the former injury site is the first body part to act up when the person is tired, stressed, or using their body improperly. In Sonia's case, her right shoulder had earlier lost its resilience to recover from abuse, and now it was acting up.

Using the Seven Commandments of Ergonomics, I performed an assessment of Sonia's work station and found that the way the equipment was set up was causing her to use her right arm at a biomechanical disadvantage.

In an ergonomic assessment of a computer work station, it's extremely important to identify the most frequent work task. Having done this, you're in a position to identify the most used piece of equipment. Next, you must assess the posture employed when the worker is using the most frequent piece of equipment: is the posture anatomically correct or is the person using excessive force to complete these repetitive tasks? Obviously the way the work station is set up affects the user's posture, and posture in turn affects both the force used to carry out the task and the need for rest breaks.

Sonia's most repetitive task, unsurprisingly, involved using her mouse, and you'll have guessed that her arm was in the wrong position when she did so. Interestingly, her arms were in the correct posture when she was using her keyboard, which was on a keyboard tray: her arms were close to her trunk and her elbows were at a 90-degree angle to the keyboard when she used it. However, when she was using her mouse with her right arm, her arm was suspended in mid-air and her elbow was straight. That's because the mouse was placed on her desktop, beside the monitor, which is by no means an unusual site.

When I used the Seven Commandments of Ergonomics checklist to perform the assessment, the majority of Sonia's equipment was correctly positioned. She had a good chair that was adjusted to *Secure the Spine*. It fit her body correctly and allowed her to sit in a perfect spinal posture. Her chair was at the correct height for her work surface and met *Beware the Chair* criteria. When using the keyboard, her elbows were aligned correctly to the keyboard, at a 90-degree angle. But half the time when she used the keyboard, she also used the mouse, and that's where the problem lay. When Sonia was using the mouse, she was working at a biomechanical disadvantage: her arm was held away from her body (in extreme range of motion), which forced the muscles of the shoulder to work overtime in order to support the weight of her arm against the effects of gravity, and it was this strain that had caused her to experience shoulder pain.

The Solution:

Sonia and I discussed the Seven Commandments of Ergonomics, and it was clear that she understood some of the basic principles involved: for instance, she had mastered the first two commandments (*Secure the Spine* and *Beware the Chair*). She understood the importance of maintaining the joints in their anatomically aligned position, but she had failed to apply this knowledge to the position of her right arm when she was mousing. Like most people, she had considered some of the ergonomic principles but not all of them. She knew enough about chairs and keyboard trays, but the mouse was an oversight. Once she was aware of where the problem lay, however, she needed no encouragement from me to make a change to her work station. Pain is a powerful motivator!

Sonia's arms were aligned perfectly when she was using her keyboard, and this was corroborated by the fact that her right shoulder was "quiet" (in other words, not painful) when she was keyboarding. That's because when she was using her keyboard, her arms were hanging loosely on each side of her trunk, and there was no muscle strain involved and no extra energy used. When she reached for the mouse, however, and especially when she reached forward in front of her body to manoeuvre the mouse, her right shoulder became what I call "nagging" immediately. To keep her shoulder quiet and protected, Sonia needed to reposition the mouse to the same height as the keyboard, which simply meant moving the mouse to the keyboard tray. Once her attention was focused so that she noticed the difference in how her right shoulder felt when using the keyboard versus when using the mouse, Sonia was more than willing to make the change.

That's when we ran into our first problem. Sonia had a standard keyboard tray that was mounted beneath the desk, and as is usually the case, her keyboard took up the entire tray, leaving no room for the mouse.

This is a very common problem in computer ergonomics, and we had several choices. We could get a longer keyboard tray, we could buy a mouse tray that would fit over the numeric keypad (Sonia didn't use that part of her keyboard anyway), or we could purchase a shorter keyboard that didn't incorporate a numeric keypad. Since I had a short keyboard with me, I asked Sonia to trial it for a week.

Without a number pad on the keyboard, there was room for the mouse on the keyboard tray. This allowed Sonia to use the mouse in a posture where reaching forward was eliminated. Her right arm was able to rest close to her body when she was mousing, and she no longer needed to reach forward with a straight elbow. Her right shoulder was now "quiet" when she was using the mouse.

When I followed up a week later, Sonia was extremely pleased with the shortened keyboard. She admitted that it had felt awkward for the first three days. Even though the short keyboard had normal-sized keys, she had still felt as though she was working in cramped quarters. But she had noticed the benefits to the shoulder almost immediately. Her right arm was now able to rest close to her body when she was mousing – no more reaching forward with a straight elbow – and her right shoulder was now "quiet" even when using the mouse. In just a week, Sonia had grown so accustomed to the short keyboard, and so delighted with the easing of her pain as a result, that she was reluctant to give it back to me. Fortunately her human resource department had already ordered her very own shortened keyboard, so I was able to wrest mine away from her without too much difficulty.

Third Commandment of Ergonomics
Align the Arms:

When I remember Sonia's problem, I think of the numerous people I see – students, office workers, commuters, and so on – who work on their computers with outstretched arms and straight elbows without experiencing any kind of discomfort. If Sonia hadn't injured her shoulder earlier in her life, would she too have been one of this fortunate group? In my mind, her former injury did predispose Sonia to a work-related injury. She also had other risk factors for such an injury: she was a woman, she was over 40 years old, she had been in the same job for over 20 years, and she participated in leisure pursuits that strained the same soft tissues that she used at work.

Another question is whether Sonia would have been receptive to making any changes to her computer work station if she hadn't been in pain. It's human nature not to change if you don't have to. If it ain't broke, why fix it? As I said above, pain is a powerful motivator; but if there's no pain, there's often little incentive to change. Most people don't stop to think that the body can take a lot of abuse before it reacts. But sooner or later, the abuse does catch up, and your discomfort slowly turns into pain.

Anatomy Lesson - Align the Arms:

Understanding the importance of using your body properly is the first step in preventing injury. Once you understand how the muscles in your arms and shoulders work, you'll understand why the third commandment concentrates on your arm posture, so here's a very short and simple anatomy lesson about how muscles move your body.

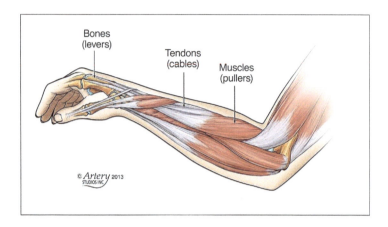

Each bone in our body is positioned beside another one, and all the bones collectively form the skeleton. When two bones are joined by ligaments, a joint is formed. Muscles act to move these joints. Muscles attach to the bones by way of tendons, which always cross a joint: one tendon attaches on one side of the joint and the other tendon attaches on the opposite side. When a muscle contracts (becomes shorter), the tendons are pulled toward each other, thus moving the bones closer together, and the joint moves. This chain reaction is called *dynamic movement*, and it's all controlled by the brain telling the body what to do. (The other form of movement is called *static* activity, and we'll discuss that in a few minutes.)

Each joint has a particular way of moving, depending on the size and shape of that joint. Remember the bones in the spine and how they stacked one on top of the other? The amount of movement that they had depended on their shape and size. Similarly, the joints in the body are also different sizes and shapes, depending on the action required.

The shoulder joint, for instance, is a ball-and-socket joint, and this allows you to move your arms in circles. The elbow, on the other hand, has a hinge type of joint, like the hinge of a door. Just as a door can close or open, the elbow can flex (like a door closing) and move your hand toward your mouth, or it can extend and straighten (like a door opening) to take your hand away from your mouth.

Therapists like me can measure the amount of movement or "range of motion" in each joint. When a joint is in its anatomically neutral or resting position, the range of motion is zero, and all the ligaments, tendons and muscles supporting that joint are working at their optimum position. When a joint is at its most stressed or most extreme range of motion, on the other hand, all the muscles and ligaments are working at their maximum exertion and are using the most energy and the most force. It's a bit like the fuel economy on a car, really. Even a Ferrari has a speed at which the engine is running at its most fuel-efficient, as well as a speed that uses so much fuel you might as well be burning twenty-dollar bills (although if you have a Ferrari, you probably didn't choose it to save gas).

But to get back to your shoulder. When your arm is hanging by your side, the soft tissues (that is, the ligaments, tendons and muscles) are working optimally. One way you know your soft tissues are working optimally is that you're not really aware of your shoulder when your arm is hanging by your side. The system is in neutral, so to speak. Now, raise your arm. Keep your elbow straight, put your hand over your head, and point your fingers to the ceiling. Hold your arm in this position for a minute. And another minute. And another minute. Are you more aware of your shoulder now? Yes, I thought you would be. Your soft tissues are working very hard to hold your arm in that position, and they're letting you know it. Your shoulder is at extreme range of motion, and your muscles are guzzling energy quickly as a result. When their energy runs out, fatigue sets in. Your shoulder gets tired and starts to feel uncomfortable. You feel a desire to drop your arm back to your side again, which is your body's way of "nagging" you to put the arm back in a position where the muscles can start recharging. Drop your arm back to its neutral posture and you'll get relief from the discomfort in your shoulder.

Desirable though it may sound to keep our bodies in a position where every joint is in its neutral state, it's really not a practical way to go through life, especially for those of us who have to earn a living. Since we can't work in a posture where every joint is positioned in its neutral state, it's important to know how to position the joints so that the soft tissues are working as close to optimum as possible. In order to avoid excessive soft tissue stress, we have to position our joints in the middle range of their movement potential.

I'd like you to think about a rubber band for a moment. (Yes, I know it's not as much fun as thinking about a Ferrari.) When the rubber band is just lying on top of your desk, empty, not stretched at all, it's at its neutral or most relaxed state. It's not working. In order for the elastic to work (by holding rolled-up pages together, for instance), it has to stretch. And the more you stretch it, the thinner it gets. If you stretch the elastic to its maximum length, it'll be at its weakest, thinnest state and could break at any minute. You may be able to stretch that rubber band to its full length a hundred times and nothing will happen, or it could break after you pull it 15 times. We can't predict its breaking point. If, however, you stretch the elastic half way (to its middle point), it'll be working at as close to optimum as possible. It's still the same width and can be used to secure whatever it is you're binding for long periods of time without breaking.

It's the same way with muscles. If you use a muscle to its most stretched position, the joint is at maximum range of motion, which means it's at its weakest and could give out in an unpredictable manner. If you use the muscle at its middle range, you can count on using it repeatedly and with strength for long periods of time. Muscles work best to move the joint when they're allowed to work as close to mid range of motion as possible.

No matter how much you may enjoy being a couch potato, the fact remains that our bodies are made to move. Energy is supplied to our muscles in terms of blood flow, which means that our muscles work best when they're moving our joints dynamically, because with dynamic movement, the blood is flowing strongly and the energy in the muscle keeps getting replenished. An example of dynamic movement would be bending your elbow to move your hand toward your face and away from it: the elbow is moving dynamically. The movement creates a pumping action, which causes surges of energy to move into your muscles. Walking is a good example of dynamic body movement. Dynamic contractions move the joints and supply energy to the muscles. Now think about this: how much dynamic muscle contraction is going on when you're working on your computer? That's right – not much. You're sitting for long periods of time with little movement occurring in your body. Your muscles are still working to hold your body upright against the effects of gravity – in fact, they're working fairly hard at this job – but they're not making your joints move. This type of muscle movement is called *static muscle contraction.*

Static muscle contraction takes a toll on our muscles because static contractions don't allow movement. When the muscle is working but not moving, the energy drains out of it quickly, and it becomes very "naggy" – that is, it's trying to attract your attention. Remember that little experiment we did in Chapter Two, where you held a pen in mid-air with your arm straight out in front of you? Remember how long you lasted before the pain got too much? Not much more than a minute, right? You were asking your shoulder muscles to work hard supporting the weight of your arm against gravity, and your shoulder soon let you know that it wasn't happy about this request.

Your shoulder started to hurt because the muscles ran out of energy, and this in turn was because there was no pumping action of the muscles to bring the energy back. Your shoulder muscles were working, but there was no movement and thus no restoration of the energy supply to them. In other words, your shoulder muscles ran out of gas.

There are hundreds of examples of the body performing static muscle contraction throughout the day in the office environment. Your muscles are working non-stop to keep you upright and erect against the forces of gravity, and every time you move out of anatomical alignment, static muscle activity occurs. Your body uses an exorbitant amount of energy daily to power all your movements, and it uses at least twice as much energy when it's struggling to hold us out of proper body alignment.

Just like Sonia, many of us are generally unaware of the fact that we're overtaxing our body when we use static muscle contraction postures. Adding to the problem is the fact that even when we do feel some pain as a result, that pain may not be in the part of our

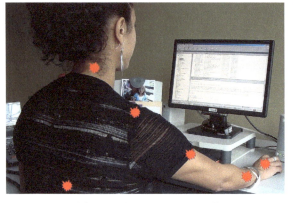

body that actually started what turned into a chain reaction. Because the muscles are so interconnected, the actions of one body part can affect many other body parts. Look at the picture of the woman working at the computer, for example. You probably spotted immediately that her right arm is in an incorrect position: in a classic example of static muscle activity of the shoulder, she's holding the arm straight when she operates her mouse. Now I'd like you to notice the red circles that give the picture such a gruesome look. Each of these circles represents a point of static muscle contraction. You can see that her incorrect arm position is affecting not only her fingers, wrist, elbow and upper arm, but also her shoulder, neck and back. A whole chain of potential problems, all stemming from the wrong position of the arm.

How to Position Your Arms to Use a Computer:

Now that you're aware of how the joints and muscles work and how to use them to the best advantage, you'll need to make sure that when you're working at your computer, you put yourself in a posture where your joints are in their neutral or resting position. It's physically impossible to work at a computer in a posture where *all* your joints are in a resting position, since typically the elbows and fingers need to be in mid range of motion if you're actually performing any real work. Here's how to achieve the best results:

Shoulders in Neutral: When your arms are directly beside your trunk, almost touching it, your shoulders are in their resting position. This is the best position for your shoulders when you're keying or mousing.

Elbows in Mid Range: The keyboard should be positioned so you can type while your arms are beside your trunk and your elbows are bent to 90 degrees. When you're using your mouse, make sure that your elbow is also positioned at 90 degrees and that your arm stays beside your body.

Arm rests: Arm rests that are useful allow you to work at forearm's distance away from the keyboard or mouse and support the forearms in a horizontal position with the elbow in a 90-degree bend. The trickiest part of getting the arm rest to fit properly is ensuring that the arms are beside the trunk when they're resting on the arm rests. Many arm rests are too wide and aren't adjusted to keep the elbows close to the trunk. Bear in mind that when your forearms are resting on the arm rests, your shoulders should be relaxed and even.

Good arm rests are made of soft material, of course, and don't have hard or sharp edges.

Placement of Tools/Equipment: Use your arms for measuring: Keeping your arms and elbows close to your trunk protects your neck, shoulders and back. That's why it's important to place your tools and/or equipment so that your most frequent tasks (more than eight times an hour) are all performed within a forearm's reach away from your body. The tasks you do occasionally (four times an hour) can be completed within arm's reach.

We're all unique and we all have different needs, so make sure all your equipment is positioned at the correct distance away from your particular body size. It's not all that complicated. If you do a lot of keyboarding, then you need to keep your arms beside your trunk, bend your elbows, and make sure your keyboard position is within forearm's reach. Your monitor should be positioned 20 to

40 centimeters or 15 to 27 inches away from your body (which translates into an arm's reach away). If you use your phone four to eight times an hour, the phone should be at arm's length as well.

Contrary to popular belief, the phone should *not* be on your dominant side. For example, if you're right handed, the phone should live on the left side of your desk. That way, when you answer the phone, you use your left hand to hold it to your ear, allowing you to use your right hand to write if necessary. This eliminates the neck flexion and extreme posture you use when you hold the phone to your ear using your shoulder and neck.

Summary:

I find it interesting that many of the people I interview at work have been assigned work stations that were previously used by someone else, yet they don't adjust the chairs or position of the equipment to fit their own body size. I don't know why! They just don't adjust the chair, change the keyboard, or move the monitor. I've worked with people who have used the same work station for over 10 years and have never changed a thing. And they often don't recognize the clues their body is giving them at the end of the work day. Be aware of that nagging body part!

Like Sonia with her frozen shoulder, we've all experienced injuries outside of the workplace. As we age, these types of injuries will be the first to resurface and cause us problems *at* the workplace. That's when we need to follow Sonia's example and listen to what our body is telling us so that we can take our cue from it. We don't, however, need to follow her example and give up our fun activities so that we can keep working. Using a computer doesn't mean that we need to experience pain at the end of the work day, nor does it mean that we need to sacrifice our leisure activities in order to work comfortably or to stay in our jobs. We can protect ourselves at work.

Our bodies are a marvel in terms of how they're made and how they move. Once we understand how our systems are interconnected, we can use this information to set ourselves up properly at work. As we've seen, our bony structures are connected by soft tissues that position and move our body. Most of the discomfort we experience at work is because we've positioned our body improperly at our work station and are unknowingly using pain-causing static muscle contraction to fight gravity. We need to position ourselves so that the bony structures and soft tissues are in their neutral or mid range. This will eliminate the static muscle contractions associated with improper posture and will prevent discomfort and pain.

The *Align the Arms* commandment looks at the structure of the arms and shows us that specifically, we need to position our shoulders and elbows in a correct posture in order to prevent or get rid of any shoulder, arm, neck, or back discomfort. This is very easy to do once you're sitting properly in your chair and your chair is correctly situated to your work station. Simply put, when you *Align the Arms*, your arms will be beside your trunk, almost touching it, and your elbows will be at a 90-degree angle. The computer keyboard will be at your fingertips. The mouse will be at your fingertips. The monitor will be an arm's length away. Congratulations on setting yourself up correctly to carry out the third ergonomic commandment!

Chapter Four

Commandment Four

Watch the Wrist

Case History:

The Problem:

Carl, age 45, had been a taxi driver for 11 years before deciding to switch to a desk job as a taxi coordinator or "call taker". As a call taker, he had to work with the telephone and the computer simultaneously. He wore a headset so that when customers called to order a cab, he could ask them for details such as their address, the time they wanted to be picked up, and their destination, and could enter the data into the computer while still talking to the customer. Between telephone calls, Carl scheduled the drivers for their shifts and reviewed the daily run sheets, checking each driver's name against the cab numbers assigned. He had worked as a call taker for five years before he finally sought medical assistance.

Carl's symptoms had actually come to his attention two years earlier, in the form of what he described as "funny" sensations in his left hand. It wasn't long, however, before the vague "funny" sensation became a definite numbness in the fingers of that hand. Since he wasn't actually in pain, Carl postponed going to the doctor. A few months later, he admitted to his wife that his fingers felt swollen now and his grip felt weak when picking up a full cup of coffee. Still, he continued to put off making an appointment to see his doctor. He did start to reconsider several months later, when his condition had deteriorated to the point where the pain in his hand woke him up five or ten times a night. But it wasn't until he woke up one night with the realization that his whole hand was numb and painful that Carl finally went to the doctor.

Carl's doctor diagnosed carpal tunnel syndrome and gave him wrist splints and pain medication. He recommended that Carl take time off work to settle his symptoms, and he stressed the importance of having an ergonomic assessment of his computer work station when Carl did return to work.

Carl took his doctor's advice, and an appointment was made for me to see him on his first day back at work. By this point, Carl was eager to work with me. He had been anxious to return to his job because he enjoyed the camaraderie he shared with the taxi drivers, missed the quick pace of the office, and frankly needed the money.

I explained the Seven Commandments of Ergonomics to him and began my assessment. Like you, Carl quickly understood that in an ergonomic assessment of a computer work station, it's extremely important to identify the most commonly performed work tasks in order to determine the effects of these repetitive tasks, the forces used in performing them, and how posture affects both the repetitive task and the force needed. So he wasn't surprised when I looked at the position of his most frequently used tools and observed his posture when he was using them.

Carl's work posture was actually quite interesting. His work station was a very old (not antique), very big wooden desk, and instead of using the back support of the chair, he sat in a forward slouch with both elbows resting on his desk. His feet dangled, so he was using a plastic milk crate for a foot rest, unaware of the fact that this positioned his knees higher than his hips.

Carl's most frequently used tools were the telephone, the keyboard and the mouse. All of these items were on his desktop, of course, but the telephone was the piece of equipment that was farthest away from him. He wore a head set, but when he answered the phone, he still had to stretch his arm forward and lift it upward to depress buttons in order to receive the call. When he wasn't answering phones, Carl sat at his desk and leaned on both elbows while performing his scheduling and checking duties on the computer. He did his job duties slouched forward while supporting the full weight of his arms on his desk.

When entering the data into the computer, Carl used the keyboard, of course, but he did so while leaning on his elbows and reaching down to strike the keys, which meant that his wrists bent backwards and forwards repeatedly as he typed. Since carpal tunnel syndrome is linked to both repeated movements of the wrist and repeated pressure to the wrist, it was easy to pinpoint the source of Carl's wrist irritation: his wrists were used in such a way that the joints were held in awkward postures and traveled through their extreme range of motion, which necessitated excessive forces to move the wrist and caused damage to the supporting soft tissues (please see previous chapter for explanation of joint range of motion).

Carl's job was an extremely busy one, with a constant stream of incoming phone calls. And for long periods every day, he slouched with both elbows on his desk, working at a frenzied pace, his wrists moving thousands of times a day as he typed rapidly, accurately, and unwisely, in a position of mechanical disadvantage. Carl worked this way for five years before his body rebelled to the point where he couldn't ignore it. Like most people, Carl ignored the early clue that something was wrong – the "funny" feeling in his hands – because he just didn't think about that symptom in the context of an injury. To Carl's way of thinking, since he wasn't lifting or carrying heavy objects, how could he suffer from a work-related injury? Meanwhile, however, his repeated wrist movements were combining with the incorrect mechanics at his wrists to increase the forces that would ultimately result in him experiencing just that fate.

The Solution:

The good news is that once you discover what's causing your discomfort or pain, you can intervene to fix the problem. Even with a diagnosis as unpleasant as carpal tunnel syndrome, all is not lost. Assisting Carl to work more comfortably involved starting with the first three commandments of computer ergonomics in order to properly achieve the fourth one – *Watch the Wrist*. Achieving ergonomic correctness involves a series of steps: it's a system that builds one step on top of the other. The main goal for any ergonomic intervention is to re-position the equipment so the person can work in a posture that's correct. To reach that goal, one must look at the spine, the arms and the wrists. In Carl's case, ensuring that his wrists were straight and in correct anatomical alignment was crucial. But we couldn't start with his wrists; we had to take care of his spinal alignment first. If you don't start by securing the spine, you can't position the wrist correctly. And as you know from previous chapters, everything depended on the position of the tools Carl used most frequently while he worked.

Starting with *Secure the Spine*, Carl thought his chair was just fine. He'd been using it for a long time and had grown accustomed to how it felt – in fact, he'd even have told you that it was comfortable. He was quite oblivious to the fact that the chair didn't provide adequate support to his spine, which was probably what had encouraged him to slouch in the first place. Specifically, the seat depth was too long, which meant that Carl sat forward in his chair so that his knees could hang over the edge of the seat. The back rest wasn't adjustable, which meant that the chair didn't support his low back curve, leaving his muscles to do all the work instead. And the arm rests were too long, which meant that he couldn't pull the chair close to the desk. No wonder he slouched!

Moving to *Beware the Chair*, we had to consider the placement of his tools. It was immediately evident that these were placed too high in relation to his arms: Carl's desk was 31 inches high, a height that effectively precluded his arms and wrists being properly aligned when he was sitting on a chair. To add to the problem, he kept his keyboard on the top of the desk instead of on a keyboard tray, which meant that it wasn't just a little too high; it was a *lot* too high for him to access correctly. Carl had raised his chair to its full height not long after he started working there, but it was still too low for the desk height, and this was another reason for his forward slouch, his habit of resting his elbows on his desk, and his need to prop his feet on a milk crate.

The third thing working against him was the position of the telephone. You remember that he used the phone on a constant basis as part of his job, right? So logically, you'd think that he'd keep it handy. However, the alert reader will recall that Carl's telephone was the tool that was farthest away from him. This hadn't seemed important to him at the time because he was given a headset, but in order to answer telephone calls, Carl had to reach his right arm to its full length to answer the phone. This, of course, meant that his arm was frequently at extreme range of motion, as was his wrist, and as we discussed in the previous chapter of this book, when a joint is at extreme range of motion, it's at a stressed position where all the muscles and ligaments are taxed to their greatest reserve. Not a good plan.

Now that we'd analyzed the problem, we had to implement the solution. The first step to help Carl was to ensure correct posture (see *Secure the Spine*). The second step was making sure that his chair matched the work height (see *Beware the Chair*). The third step was ensuring he could work in a posture where he didn't have to reach: in other words, a posture where his arms were resting beside his trunk (see *Align the Arms*). And the fourth step – the most crucial one, in this case – was to ensure proper anatomical alignment of the wrist: that is, to *Watch the Wrist*.

A new chair was purchased that matched Carl's size and his workplace needs. It had an adjustable back rest that we positioned to support his low back; it had shorter arm rests that allowed him to sit close to his work surface; and it was able to be raised so that he could access the tools on his desk surface from the correct height and without stretching. In addition, Carl's old plastic milk crate was honourably retired to the nearest recycling centre, and a proper foot support was installed so that his knees and hips were at 90 degrees when he was sitting. Once the chair was set up and adjusted to his spine, we placed it in front of the computer. The keyboard and the phone, which Carl used simultaneously and constantly, were repositioned on the desk surface so that they were within forearm's length instead of requiring him to reach to arm's length to use them. This repositioning allowed his upper arms to hang beside his trunk, with the weight of the arms supported by the arm rests of the chair. All was now right with Carl's work station: he was sitting with his spine aligned, his chair had been adjusted so his arms were close to his body and his elbow was bent at 90 degrees, and his equipment had been moved to the edge of the desk and positioned at an angle where his wrists were anatomically neutral.

But humans are creatures of habit. After the ergonomic adjustments had been made, Carl reported that he felt awkward. In particular, he didn't feel comfortable with the new position of his equipment, insisting that it felt too close to his body. I couldn't really blame him for feeling that way. After all, he'd been working in a slouched posture with both elbows on the desk for more than five years, so it was quite understandable that the new setup would feel awkward at first. I asked him to try the adjustments for a one-week period, and although he hesitated at first, when I gently reminded him that the ergonomic assessment had been recommended by his doctor, he agreed to give it a try.

Reluctant Carl may have been, but he kept an open mind, and on follow-up a week later, he reported that he felt much better. He told me happily that he was sleeping through the night now and was able to do his job with more energy. He even confided that his back pain and shoulder discomfort had been reduced to the point of being "insignificant" – which was especially interesting to me because this was the first time he'd mentioned problems with his back and shoulder! I felt that this was a breakthrough for Carl and a great example of the benefits and importance of the seven ergonomic commandments, demonstrating that a systematic intervention to correct a person's working posture can help not only the problems the therapist knows about but even the ones she doesn't. For a moment there, I felt almost like a magician.

Fourth Commandment of Ergonomics

Watch the Wrist:

Carl's case confirms that ergonomic intervention isn't always straightforward. When implementing ergonomic changes, you may have to change more than one thing to fix the actual problem; it's like a chain reaction. With Carl, we had to intervene with the chair first before we could start to eliminate the wrist pain. What's needed is a systematic way to look at problems at the workplace so that you can analyze *all* the factors involved and then make the necessary changes to increase your comfort and decrease your pain. With a system like the Seven Commandments of Ergonomics, you can work step by step in the correct sequence so that all factors are covered. The correct time to implement the fourth commandment, for example, is when the other three commandments have been put into practice. You must be sitting with your spine aligned properly (*Secure the Spine*), your chair adjusted specifically to your work space (*Beware the Chair*), and your elbows bent at 90 degrees, with your most frequently used piece of equipment at your fingertips (*Align the Arms*). Only then are you ready to move on to the next commandment (*Watch the Wrist*).

I believe that if you understand the mechanics of your wrist and know *why* it's important to position it in an anatomically correct position, the fourth commandment will make more sense to you. Please read the brief anatomy lesson below; I've done my best to keep it simple.

Anatomy Lesson – Watch The Wrist:

The main job of your wrist is to position your hand for the many different functions it performs – holding, squeezing, pinching, precision work, etc. The wrist is an amazing collection of bones, joints and soft tissues that all work together so you can interact with your environment. It provides the fulcrum for movement of the hand, and it helps the hand to stabilize objects and to generate force or strength. Let's take a look at the bones and soft tissues that comprise the wrist, so that we can better understand the importance of keeping them in their correct anatomical position when working. Once you understand the wrist, you'll understand our susceptibility to those three words feared by all keyboardists – carpal tunnel syndrome.

The wrist itself is made up of eight small bones that link your forearm at one end to your fingers at the other. In other words, the wrist connects your arm to your hand. The eight bones touch each other, and at each point of intersection, a joint is formed. These joints are attached to each other by ligaments. Ligaments provide stability for the joints; muscles provide movement (they attach to the bones by way of tendons). Movement of the joints, and hence movement of the hand, is made possible by muscle contractions.

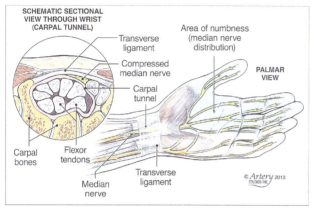

The small bones of the wrist, called carpal bones, are positioned by the ligaments to join together and form a narrow horseshoe shape. The horseshoe has an open end, of course, and you can see in the illustration that there's a band of ligament (called the transverse ligament) that acts as a roof and closes the horseshoe. In doing so, this ligament in essence creates a tunnel: yes, the dreaded carpal tunnel. It's through this tunnel that the median nerve passes, as do the nine flexor tendons.

The median nerve is very important for the hand. It allows your hand to feel and most (but not all) of your fingers to move, and it carries messages to your brain so that your brain tells your hand what to do, and how and where to move. It sends messages to the brain about what the hand is feeling: for example, heat or cold, softness or hardness. Your brain needs to know that information so that it can tell the hand how to respond.

The tendons are important too, because they attach the muscles to the bones, and it's the muscles that actually allow your hand to move. So we have one important nerve and nine important tendons passing through the carpal tunnel – which, I might point out, is only about as big as your index finger. Obviously any interference within this tiny space in the carpal tunnel is going to interfere with the function, feeling and movement of the hand. In particular (as again you can see from the illustration), it's going to interfere with the pain-free usefulness of the thumb, the index finger, the middle finger, and (somewhat improbably) only the half of the ring finger that's closest to the thumb.

What can happen to interfere with the carpal tunnel? Well, since the space in the carpal tunnel is so small, any swelling or thickening of the structures that pass through it can cause problems. And what might cause this swelling or thickening? Unfortunately, just about any injury or irritation can cause inflammation to any of the soft tissues that pass through the tunnel, and with inflammation comes swelling. If the tendons that pass through the tunnel become irritated by too much movement, for example, the resultant swelling may cause them to press on the nerve that also passes through the tunnel. If that happens, it causes pain, weakness, or numbness in the hand and wrist. The ligaments too can get irritated by the swollen tendons, and this would similarly cause increased pressure in the tunnel, with much the same result: pain, weakness, or numbness.

As in Carl's case, symptoms of carpal tunnel problems usually start gradually. The first clues are signs of discomfort. Some people report that their fingers feel thick and swollen, or that they burn or tingle. Some even report a kind of itching numbness. The discomfort usually starts in the dominant hand, which of course is the hand that's used most often during the day.

Bearing in mind the structure of the wrist and especially the carpal tunnel setup, you can easily see why performing the same hand and wrist movements on a repetitive basis leads to carpal tunnel syndrome. Incidentally, jobs that require pinching, gripping and/or working with the wrist bent are the ones with the highest incidence of the syndrome. The people most prone to carpal tunnel syndrome are checkout clerks in grocery stores, assembly line workers, carpenters, meat packers, violinists, mechanics, people who use vibrating equipment (jackhammers, for example), and – of course – people who use computers. I find it interesting that women between the ages of 40 and 60 are three times more likely to develop carpal tunnel syndrome. If you fit into one or more of these categories, please pay close attention to the fourth commandment of ergonomics – *Watch the Wrist*. (Of course, if you're a 50-year-old female who uses a jackhammer by day, plays the violin at night, and spends her weekends doing carpentry, you may be beyond help!)

Treatment for carpal tunnel syndrome includes rest (or changing how you use your hand – yes, it really is true that sometimes a change is as good as a rest), a wrist brace, medication, and sometimes surgery. Putting ice on your wrist, massaging the area, and/or doing stretching exercises of the wrist may help too. Of course, carpal tunnel syndrome isn't the only cause of wrist pain, so please consult with your doctor if you have discomfort or pain in your wrist. An ergonomic assessment of your work station will be important if you're going to change how you use your hands.

A wrist brace can work in the same way as an ergonomic assessment, to some extent. The goal is the same, but the methods of achieving it are different. An ergonomic assessment will analyze the flaws in your work station and suggest adjustments that will allow your wrist to be in a neutral position when you work, whereas the brace (if it fits properly) locks your wrist in its neutral position and thus helps to support the carpal tunnel in anatomically correct alignment. Since the carpal tunnel is at its widest when in this neutral position, the median nerve and all the structures that pass through the tunnel are at their least compressed. The philosophy of the brace is thus to maintain the carpal tunnel at its greatest diameter when the wrist is at rest. On the other hand, the philosophy of the fourth commandment – *Watch the Wrist* – is to maintain the carpal tunnel at its greatest diameter when the wrist is working. Whichever way you go about it, I believe the best work practice is to make sure your wrist is in its anatomically neutral position when working. The best cure is always prevention!

How to Position your Wrist to Use a Computer:

*W*atch the Wrist. You must make sure that your wrist is in its proper anatomical position if you're going to ensure a neutral wrist posture when you're working at your computer. Those of you who've read about the shape and size of the bones in our body can appreciate how the bones fit together, and also how the soft tissues work most effectively when the joints are aligned. Here are the steps to ensure that you work with your wrists in neutral.

1. **Use Landmarks to Make Sure Your Wrists are Aligned Properly:** I want to introduce you to some landmarks that will guide you to position your wrist in its anatomically neutral and correct position.

   a) <u>Thumb and Forearm</u>. When the thumb and the forearm are in a straight line, the wrist is in a perfectly aligned position.

   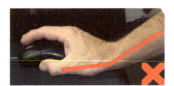 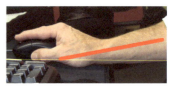

   Self-Check: The alignment of the wrist to your most used piece of equipment is of the utmost importance. To make sure your wrist is in a neutral position, place the entire length of your forearm – from the elbow to the finger tips – on your desk top, with the palm facing the table.

   Pretend you're cupping an orange. Now look at the back of your hand. Your knuckles will look as if they're bent slightly backwards. This is okay as it's the natural arch of your hand. Now look at your thumb. Notice how it's lined up with your forearm; the thumb should be aligned at

12 o'clock with the forearm. Lock your wrist in that position. It's the position your wrist should be in when you're working, if you want to make sure that those important soft tissues passing through your carpal tunnel aren't compromised. Memorize it!

b) <u>Knuckle and Forearm</u>. Now look at the back of your hand again. The third knuckle should be centred on your forearm.

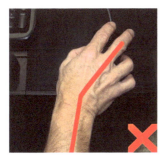 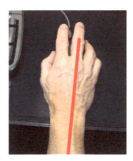

When you have these two landmarks aligned, your wrist is in its correct anatomical posture and the carpal tunnel is at its greatest diameter. With your wrist in this position, there's minimal pressure on the structures that run through the tunnel.

2. **Avoid Contact Pressure to Your Wrists:** When you're typing on your keyboard, your wrists shouldn't be resting on a wrist support or a hard surface, no matter what the nice salesman in the computer store told you. Your wrists should be floating, the way a piano player's wrists do. (Some piano teachers make you practise scales while balancing a pencil on the back of the hand, so as to keep the wrists and hands in the correct position. Try that exercise sometime when you're typing!) When you stop entering data – let's say you're thinking about what aspect you should tackle next, for instance – *that's* when your wrists can rest on a wrist support.

Remember, you want to avoid increasing the pressure on the carpal tunnel. In order to do this, the wrist rest should be wider than one and a half inches to avoid excessive pressure.[xi]

When resting your hand on the wrist rest, it's the base of your palm that should be resting there, not your forearm!

Hint: Some keyboards have legs on the back, in order to let you tilt the unit to make the row of number keys higher than the row with the space bar. This may sound as if it would be more comfortable, but in fact it can cause you to work with the wrist in an extended (bent backward) and incorrect position. Take care not to allow the angle of the keyboard to cause your wrist to bend either backward or forward.

Summary:

It's not the "all of a sudden" types of things that cause injury at the computer. The types of actions that cause computer-related injury are the common, unspectacular things that we do every working day. On their own, those actions involve little to no danger, but when combined with other things, they can become very risky indeed in terms of possible injuries.

Performing the same hand and wrist movements on a repetitive basis can lead to carpal tunnel syndrome. Jobs that require pinching, gripping and/or working with the wrist bent have the highest incidence of carpal tunnel problems. Women between the ages of 40 and 60 are three times more likely to develop carpal tunnel syndrome. If you're a checkout clerk in a grocery store, an assembly line worker, a carpenter, a meat packer, a violinist, or a mechanic, you're in one of the occupations most prone to problems with carpal tunnel. Ditto if you use a computer or vibrating equipment. If you fit into these categories, please *Watch the Wrist*.

Don't be like Carl, performing the same wrist movements over and over again at a frantic pace while in a poor posture. Otherwise you'll end up like Carl, suffering from soft tissue damage as a result of causing your body to generate more force than necessary when moving your wrists as part of your job. Instead, look at your body as if it were a machine. You wouldn't expect a machine to continue working at its optimum if its parts were malaligned and used too often, now would you? So treat your body with the same respect. Don't make it use more force/energy than necessary to perform an action just because it isn't positioned properly. And if your body's "Check Engine" light starts coming on – in other words, if you experience discomfort – for goodness' sake pay attention. Don't be like Carl and ignore it.

You need a *systematic* way to look at problems at the workplace so that you analyze *all* the factors and make *all* the necessary changes to increase your comfort. The Seven Commandments of Ergonomics will help you to work one step at a time to make sure you're following the correct sequence in making the ergonomic changes that will enable you to position yourself correctly. The correct time to implement the fourth commandment is when you're sitting with your spine aligned properly, your chair adjusted specifically to the work space, and your elbows bent at 90 degrees, with your most frequently used piece of equipment at your fingertips: in other words, when the first three commandments have been satisfied.

There are two important landmarks to help you fulfil the fourth commandment and thus *Watch the Wrist*. The first landmark is related to your thumb. When you're using the keyboard or the mouse, your thumb must be aligned in a straight line with your forearm. The second landmark is your third knuckle, which must also be aligned in a straight line with the forearm.

You can use a wrist rest, but not when you're actively using the keyboard. Only use it when resting (or thinking). If you do use a wrist rest, make sure it's more than one and a half inches wide and also make sure you rest the base of your palms, not your forearm, on it.

Now you can use those landmarks to guide you on your way to a pain-free work environment.

Chapter Five

Commandment Five

Check the Chin

Case History:

The Problem:

Wendy was a 32-year-old, newly married, self-employed event coordinator who was beginning to panic – not about her business but about her fear that she wouldn't be able to fulfil her partnership commitment in her marriage. She and her husband had a wonderful relationship, but Wendy was finding that she just couldn't manage to keep working for extended periods of time any longer, and she was scared that her condition would deteriorate to the point where she wouldn't be able to work at all. How could she fulfil her partnership commitment if she couldn't work? How would they pay for their newly acquired home if they didn't have her income to add to her husband's?

Wendy had been in a car accident eight months earlier, and ever since then, she'd been unable to work comfortably. During her ergonomic evaluation, she told me she began every day with discomfort/stiffness in her neck and upper back, and it quickly worsened during the work day and turned into pain. Poor Wendy now spent so much time trying to cope with her pain that she couldn't concentrate very well on her work.

In her position as an event coordinator, she worked mostly in her home, using her laptop computer. She didn't have a designated work area within the home but carried the laptop to different locations within her house and tried to arrange herself so that she'd be comfortable.

Because Wendy worked in so many different locations, you might think that she couldn't be having the same problem in each spot, but in fact that was exactly what was happening. When I watched her using her laptop in three different places, I could easily see the common factor: she wasn't working in an ergonomically correct posture, and her seated posture revealed numerous ergonomic risk factors for injury.

You remember from previous chapters, I'm sure, that in an ergonomically correct work posture, there are anatomical landmarks that are aligned. For example, in Commandment #1, *Secure the Spine*, we learned that the correct posture ensured that the ears are directly above the shoulders, and the hips and knees are maintained at 90 degrees of flexion. In Commandment #3, *Align the Arms*, the arms must be positioned alongside the trunk, with the elbows positioned at 90 degrees. And in Commandment #4, *Watch the Wrist*, we saw that the wrist must be in neutral so the thumb is aligned with the forearm. When all these landmarks are aligned, it means your posture is correct. And no, I didn't forget Commandment #2. That's the one that told us we should take care to ensure that this correct posture is maintained by having a supportive chair at the correct work height while we're working (*Beware the Chair*). Now we're turning our attention to the fifth commandment, which relates to correct head position. For a correct head position, the chin must be directly above the sternal notch and parallel to the ground. I'll explain exactly what the sternal notch is in a minute.

In Wendy's situation, when she was using her laptop, her chin was noticeably in the wrong position. The neck and shoulder pain that she was experiencing had been initially and directly caused by the car accident six months earlier, but the incorrect position in which she was holding her head when working was aggravating that pain. When she looked at her laptop, Wendy's head was bent so far forward that her chin was almost touching her breastbone. To make matters worse, when she used the laptop, Wendy's shoulders were uneven: her shoulder blades were "winged", making the shoulders themselves rounded, so that she looked as if she were sitting in a slouched, hunchbacked posture.

I see many people working in this type of hunched posture when using a laptop, and most of them don't report any problems associated with the position. Wendy herself had worked in this posture for years with no problems, so why was she having pain now? Well, when she was in the car accident, Wendy had suffered whiplash-type soft tissue injuries. She hadn't broken any bones, but she had strained her muscles and they hadn't fully recovered yet. Her body, still struggling to recuperate from those injuries, could no longer cope with the subtle abuse caused by working in a poor posture. Remember, computer-related injuries don't happen all of a sudden. They develop over time, slowly and innocently, and as you've seen, they're definitely related to poor posture. In the silent epidemic of the 90s, it took approximately 10 years of computer use before injuries began to be reported, but in Wendy's case, the injuries from her car accident caused her body to rebel against its poor working posture in a matter of weeks, not years.

The Solution:

Again, as with any ergonomic intervention, implementing the Seven Commandments of Ergonomics means that you follow the commandments in sequence; they were designed to be a step-by-step process. Identify the most commonly performed work task, start with Commandment #1 (*Secure the Spine*), and then move through the commandments in numerical order. Although Wendy's most obvious problem related to her incorrect head position when using the laptop, we couldn't solve this problem unless we first dealt with the other postural mistakes that were contributing to the incorrect head posture. Wendy's problems were two-fold: she had both a sore back and a sore neck, and they quickly became painful when she tried to work.

The first thing I wanted to do was to support Wendy's neck and back at the same time. Fortunately, I spied a reclining chair in her living room. It turned out that her husband used it when he was watching television. I put Wendy in the recliner, and we tilted it half-way back so that her head was supported by the recliner's pillow. Naturally this took all the strain off her head and neck. It eliminated not only the forward bend of her head but also all the static muscle contraction that had been occurring in her neck, shoulders and upper back muscles. The bonus was that the back rest of the recliner had a built-in low back support which fit the contours of Wendy's low back perfectly. So we had accomplished Commandment #1, *Secure the Spine*. We then moved on through the rest of the commandments, keeping in mind that *Check the Chin* was of the utmost importance.

While Wendy was resting in the chair in a reclined position, our goal was to keep her head in supported alignment while satisfying all seven of the commandments. (Don't worry, I know that we've only reached Commandment #5 so far.) In order to keep her head in supported alignment, we had to raise the laptop computer into Wendy's visual field while she was reclining. We did this by placing one of her decorative pillows on her lap and then putting the laptop on top of the pillow. She was now able to see the laptop monitor without changing the position of her head. With her laptop on the pillow, her arms were naturally positioned beside her trunk and her elbows were at 90 degrees to the keyboard. Her wrists were in neutral. Mission accomplished! All of the first five ergonomic commandments had been met! Wendy was thrilled with these temporary measures.

There was, however, one other problem. Since her car accident, Wendy couldn't sit in one spot for long periods of time: she became too stiff. She now knew that sitting in the recliner would allow her to use the laptop without added pain, but she asked for another work area as well. This request was more challenging, but I like a good challenge.

Prowling around Wendy's home in search of another area that she could work comfortably in, I peered into her husband's office and noticed an antique desk with a matching antique wooden chair that had a straight back made of spindles. Wendy assured me that the desk was mainly for decorative purposes and that her husband would be happy for her to utilize it. All that was needed to transform this into an alternative work station was a little creativity on my part. As always, I started with the first commandment, *Secure the Spine*, and then I began working my way toward the fifth one, *Check the Chin*.

How do you *Secure the Spine* when using a straight-backed old wooden chair? That's where the creativity came in. I found out that Wendy had recently purchased a support cushion for her low back (she planned to use it when driving), and we were able to fit this lumbar support into the chair at the correct height to support her low back curve. But that was just the beginning. Next we had to match the height of the chair to the height of the desk. This meant we had to position the laptop so that Wendy's arms were beside her body and her elbows were bent to 90 degrees when she was using it. More inventiveness was clearly called for! We began by pulling open the top drawer of the desk and resting the laptop on the edge of the drawer. The good news was that the laptop was now at the correct height, but the bad news was that it fell backwards into the drawer at the slightest provocation. To stop this from happening, we put a phone book in the drawer to fill up the empty space, and this held the laptop level.

These somewhat unconventional adaptations allowed Wendy to be positioned in an ergonomically correct head posture. How did I know? Because her chin was now parallel to the floor and above her sternal notch. (I told you we'd come back to the sternal notch, didn't I?) This is the next anatomical landmark I'd like you to get familiar with. The sternal notch is part of your breastbone, so go ahead and put your hand on your breastbone. Now move your hand along the breastbone and toward your head, until you get to the very top of the breastbone (you'll be at the soft part of your throat). Now press a little harder. Feel the bony notch there? That's your sternal notch. When working, your chin should always be over that notch. Why? The answer is in the anatomy lesson below. Remember, these anatomy lessons are very simple explanations, giving you just enough information to make sure you understand how your body works and what you need to do so that your body can use the computer effortlessly and without pain.

Fifth Commandment of Ergonomics
Check the Chin:

Anatomy Lesson:

In *Secure the Spine* (Chapter 1), we learned about the vertebrae that collectively form the backbone or spine. Do you remember that the spine consists of a series of uniquely shaped bones called vertebrae? You might remember, then, that their size and shape vary depending on what part of the back they're found in. The seven vertebrae in the neck, for instance, are smaller and flatter than those in the trunk or low back. That's because the head sits on, and is moved by, the neck. The head has many different planes of movement: we can look up at the ceiling (extension), we can look down at the floor (flexion), we can look beside us (rotation), and we can bend our ear toward our shoulders (lateral flexion). It's the size and shape of the vertebrae in our neck that allows our head to move in all of these directions.

One thing that I didn't address in Chapter 2, however, is the soft tissues that support the vertebrae. Bones (like the vertebrae, for example) are hard, and they provide our body with rigidity, which allows us to stand straight. However, totally rigid bodies wouldn't be able to move; hence whenever two bones meet, we have muscle attachments at the resulting joint to allow for mobility. Unlike bones, muscles are considered to be "soft tissue". Another important soft tissue structure is the disc, as in "slipped disc". In between each of the vertebrae in our neck and back are discs (technically known as intervertebral discs) that separate the bones and act as a shock absorber by providing a cushion between them.

I'm told that a healthy disc has the consistency of crab meat. In

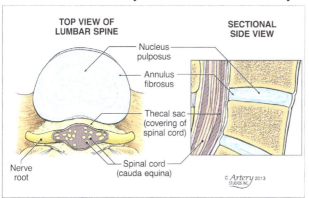

appearance, the disc resembles an onion in that the outer portion of the disc (known as the annulus fibrosus) consists of 15 to 25 concentric sheets of collagen (called the lamellae) that look just like the layers of an onion. This layered portion has a jelly-like nucleus at its centre, called the nucleus pulposus. (This section is starting to sound like a cook book, isn't it? Crab meat, onions, and now jelly.)

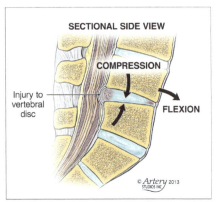

SECTIONAL SIDE VIEW

COMPRESSION

Injury to vertebral disc

FLEXION

© *Artery* 2013
STUDIOS INC.

Obviously when you stand, there is pressure on all the discs that separate the bony vertebrae of the neck and back. The pressure exerted on these discs is constant because the discs are constantly holding up the weight of the body against the force of gravity. As long as you stand in an anatomically correct posture, this pressure is evenly distributed across the disc, and the outer layers and the nucleus remain the same height because the evenness of the pressure allows the jelly-like nucleus to maintain its original shape. When the body bends forward, however, there's more pressure on the front part of the disc, which naturally causes the front layers of the disc to flatten, which in turn causes the nucleus to bulge backwards, which pushes the layers of the annulus (the "onion") toward the back of the disc. Over time, you can imagine what happens. The backward movement of the nucleus starts to fray the layers of the annulus, and the nucleus itself starts to leak out through the ensuing gaps. Once all the layers are sufficiently frayed, the disc is ruptured and the nucleus can escape, at which point it presses on the surrounding soft tissues of the body that are now in its way. That probably doesn't sound very dramatic ("Help, help! My nucleus pulposus has escaped!" isn't a line you're likely to find in any scary movie), but believe me, the pain is excruciating.

Why excruciating? Let's look at the bigger picture. The bony vertebrae form a column that provides protection to the spinal cord that runs through its central cavity, and each disc lies between two vertebrae. At the level of each vertebra, the spine sends out either motor nerves or sensory nerves. These nerves are very important, because they tell our muscles either how to move (motor) or how to interpret information from the environment (sensory). They tell our brain whether things are hot or cold, soft or hard, etc. These nerves bring back information from the muscles to the brain and allow us to feel pain. (Sometimes, of course, we all wish they wouldn't do that with quite so much enthusiasm.)

What's very important to understand is that the nerves from the brain travel (in the form of the spinal cord) through the centre of the vertebrae along the entire length of the back. Specific nerves exit at different levels of the vertebrae and go to specific parts of the body so that those body parts can move or have sensation. And if a ruptured disc presses against one of the nerves that exit the vertebrae at any level, the pain is agonising to the point where it has caused people to become bedridden. It's described as feeling like electric shocks, or like tingling and numbness, and it can also be associated with muscle weakness. If this intense pain is in the low back area, it can even cause bowel and bladder problems. Incidentally, although the most common site for a ruptured disc is in the low back area, the pain itself may actually occur in your buttock and leg because that's the region of the body that those exiting nerves travel to.

Although disc rupture is far less common in the neck, the nerves that supply our arms are the ones that exit the vertebrae at the neck (cervical spine), and thus arm discomfort can be related to the position you hold your head in when you work. And arm discomfort isn't the only problem that can result from incorrect head posture. Not only can you experience neck pain caused by soft tissue strain resulting from poor head posture, but things will get more complicated when that soft tissue strain is combined with disc bulging and/or what's known as nerve impingement: that is, when a misalignment of one or more of the joints in the spine places pressure on a nerve. Those factors can add a headache to the mix, and/or you may experience pain, weakness, or even loss of sensation in the shoulder muscles or chest.

In other words, poor neck posture causing uneven pressure distribution on the intervertebral discs of the cervical spine can eventually affect how you use a *lot* of different parts of your upper body.

And that's why it's so important to *Check the Chin* (Commandment #5) when you're working at your computer: because when your chin is in the anatomically correct position (with your chin parallel to the floor and over your sternal notch), then the vertebrae are aligned, the pressure on the discs in your neck is evenly distributed, and there's less wear and tear on the discs and therefore less likelihood of a disc bulge, a rupture, or pressure on a nerve. This position is also easier on the muscles that work to support your head against the effects of gravity: it's the position that allows them to work while expending the least amount of energy.

How do you Check the Chin?

Here's a step-by-step method to ensure you meet Commandment #5. Following these steps will help you to work in a correct chin position, provided you don't need to wear progressive lenses when you work.

Step 1: Chin over the sternal notch: Your chin should be directly over your sternal notch. To find your sternal notch, touch your breastbone (sternum), then run your fingers up toward your head until you come to the hollow in your neck. Press firmly and you'll feel a bony notch. When you're working, your chin should be directly above this notch: not to the right of it, not to the left of it, but directly over the top of it.

To keep your head in this position, you may need to reposition your monitor, because that's the piece of equipment that's crucial to chin position. If your monitor was a mirror, your nose would be in the centre of it.

Step 2: Chin parallel to the floor: When working, your chin alignment should run parallel to the floor. Typically, the way to check this is to make sure that the tool bar on your computer monitor is at the same height as your eyebrows. This tends to position your chin parallel to the floor. To adjust the tool bar to the same height as your eyebrows, just raise or lower your monitor.

Step 3. Mid range of head movement: In the real world, of course, you won't always be able to keep your chin parallel to the floor or your head over your sternal notch when you're working, because you'll need to move your head to look at other things at your work station, such as hard copy. In those circumstances, you need to use middle range of motion. (Check Chapter 2 to refresh your memory, if you've forgotten this rule.) Remember, your muscles use the least amount of energy when in their anatomically correct position, and we want our muscles to be relaxed and happy, don't we? So the goal is to stay within your chin's inner to mid range of movement, which would be up to 30 degrees of head movement. That applies to looking sideways *and* to looking down.

How can you accomplish this? If you need to refer to hard copy, then position the hard copy to either side of your monitor or else directly below it. Make sure your hard copy is on an inclined surface and not flat on the desk.

If you're using a laptop, raise it so that your chin isn't flexed forward more than 30 degrees. A portable laptop stand is ideal for this type of situation. You can buy one of the models that are available commercially or, if you're the ingenious type, you can create your own. I have, on numerous occasions, raised the height of my laptop so that the screen is at the appropriate height for a monitor, and then plugged in a separate keyboard that I've used at a lower height in order to make the work station ergonomically correct.

Multiple Monitors: During my ergonomic wanderings, I'm finding that more and more offices have work stations with more than one monitor. A frequent question is where to position the monitors so that the chin remains over the sternal notch. The answer is easy! Which monitor is used most frequently? That's the one that should be centred, with the other monitor(s) placed within a visual field that doesn't exceed 30 degrees of chin position out of neutral. If there are two monitors that are used with almost equal frequency, then the central point should be where these monitors intersect.

If you use two monitors, they should be positioned an arm's reach away. If you use three monitors at a time, they need to be positioned further away than arm's reach, so that your eye muscles can accommodate to the multiple screens.

Glare: Whereas glare on a computer screen was a significant problem in days past, most monitors now have low reflective screens, and I only occasionally run into this problem. To avoid glare and the awkward head positions that accompany glare problems, here are some hints:

- Avoid placing your computer in front of a window. If you can't avoid working in front of the window, then position your computer at a 90-degree angle to it. And if you can't do *that*, I'm sorry, but you may have to close the blinds.

- If you have fluorescent lighting in the office, position the computer screen at a parallel line with the tubing. You may also have to shut off the lights in the hallways to eliminate glare.

- Use indirect lighting, making sure the light illuminates the document and not the monitor.

- Use an anti-glare screen or hood.

Progressive Lenses:

When you're in your 40s, you usually can't see objects clearly at close range with the naked eye. (The good news is that this makes it harder for you to see the laugh lines as they start making themselves at home.) There are several possible solutions for this change in visual acuity, all of them involving glasses of one sort or another.

Let's start with progressive lenses. These are glasses that are claimed to work for everything: that is, they're said to allow for clear vision at all distances from near (16 inches) to far (20 feet). I have some of these glasses myself, but unfortunately I find they don't work well for computer use. The problem with progressive lens is that the intermediate zone of the lens is also the narrowest zone, and it's hard to stay in this focal zone when you're using the computer. Once my gaze drifts outside of this zone, there seems to be distortion when I'm trying to focus on the computer screen.

Then there are general purpose bifocals, but in my experience and observation, these are also difficult to use comfortably with a computer. I've seen many instances where the wearer of progressive lenses or bifocals tilts their head back in order to improve their focus on the monitor while looking through the lower segment of the lenses. While it may help them to see the screen more clearly, such a backward tilt of the head breaks the fifth ergonomic commandment, Check the Chin, by taking the chin out of a parallel alignment with the floor. The result is that this posture puts excessive pressure on the soft tissue in the neck, especially the cervical discs, thus leading to neck and shoulder pain and possibly arm and low back pain as well.

So instead of changing the position of your chin, change the position of the monitor: lower it until the tool bar is lower than your eyebrows, and in some instances, much lower. You'll have to experiment to find the correct height for you and your particular lens, but when you find the spot that you think is right, be sure to ask a co-worker to check that when you're viewing the screen through the lower part of your glasses, your chin is parallel to the floor.

Single vision lenses are much better for computer use than bifocals and progressive lenses are. However, bifocals can be adapted so that the upper segment is set up for the distance from the monitor while the lower segment is set up for work that's closer than the computer screen (i.e., reading distance). The drawback is that objects farther away than the monitor are blurry, but perhaps your colleagues look better in soft focus.

Progressive lenses can also be changed to have a larger area for mid-distance use, and this set-up normally provides the most comfort. These types of lenses are typically referred to as occupational progressive lenses. They provide the wearer with full-width viewing for the display distance (that is, the monitor) as well as full-width viewing for reading. The drawback is that they don't have distance vision. Unfortunately, mixing glasses with computer monitors is one of those situations where you just can't have it all.

Summary:

Following the Seven Commandments for Computer Ergonomics makes sense when you understand the way the body is built and how it works. The Commandment #5, Check the Chin, was extremely important to Wendy after she was involved in a car accident and sustained soft tissue injuries to her neck and back.

Bones provide our body with rigidity, while soft tissues support or move the bones. The bones in the neck (called vertebrae) are of a certain size and are shaped a certain way in order to allow the head to move in many different directions. The vertebrae protect the spinal cord: they form a column with a central canal through which the spinal cord travels. There are discs in between the vertebrae that allow for shock absorption. At the level of each vertebra, spinal cord nerves exit the column to supply the muscles of the body with sensation or movement. There is continual wear and tear on all these structures, and this is accelerated when correct anatomical alignment isn't maintained. Awkward and extreme static postures are an indicator of poor anatomical alignment. Poor anatomical alignment causes uneven weight distribution on the intervertebral discs and can result in a ruptured disc, which is acutely painful. Because so many nerves exit the spinal cord at the neck, incorrect head position can cause pain in the neck and may also result in headaches, shoulder pain, upper back pain, arm pain, and wrist pain. In order to prevent pain, or to relieve the pain you already have, pay attention to your head position. Keep your chin parallel to the floor and directly over your sternal notch (breastbone) when working. You can accomplish this by moving your computer monitor or raising your laptop. Your goal is to have the on-screen toolbar at the same height as your eyebrows. In jobs where you work from hard copy and use a computer monitor, you'll have to position your hard copy to either side of the monitor, or directly below it, in order to keep your head in mid range of movement.

If you're more aware of your neck at the end of the work day, don't forget to *Check the Chin*.

Chapter Six

Commandment Six

Centre the Nose

Case History:

The Problem:

At the age of 55, JoAnne wasn't slowing down at all when it came to work. A lawyer with a specialty in tax law, she was also a partner in the firm, which pretty much guaranteed that her working days were at least 12 hours long. JoAnne could cope with the hours, but she was having increasing difficulty coping with the pain in her neck, shoulders and upper back, and she couldn't help noticing that it was steadily getting worse. She'd grown accustomed to a degree of ongoing discomfort in her low back area – it had been part of her life for quite some time, after all – but now that her neck and shoulders were starting to act up as well, JoAnne was worried enough to ask for an outside consultation.

As part of her law firm's business plan, all the offices were going to be re-decorated and fitted out with new furniture, so JoAnne hired me to work with the designer. She wanted to ensure that her furniture didn't just look good, she wanted it to function well and be set up in a way that would help her to get rid of her pain. JoAnne wasn't going to settle for less than the best, and I had *carte blanche* to recommend any equipment that was needed. This was quite a novelty for me, and I must admit it was very exciting. Most of my clients have to work within certain budgetary constrictions, but not JoAnne. As far as she was concerned, it was full steam ahead and hang the expense!

Even when you have *carte blanche* to buy whatever the client needs to solve the problem, though, you still have to work through the same logical steps to assess what's been causing it. So, as with all my ergonomic consultations, I reviewed her job duties and identified her most frequently performed work tasks. It was no surprise that JoAnne's most common work tasks involved using the keyboard and mouse, of course, but along with that, she frequently needed to manipulate files containing hard-copy information that she had to review and input. She also told me that she used the telephone a great deal and that her telephone calls could be quite lengthy. While on the phone, JoAnne would input data into the computer. So she had two distinctly different needs to consider – her equipment and her hard copy.

Watching the person at work is an important part of every ergonomic consultation, and while you watch the postures they use, you have to keep their complaints in the forefront of your mind. When I watched JoAnne's posture while she was working with paper, I could see right away that she had a poor head position: her head was out of alignment with her shoulders. She also didn't sit against the back of her chair, and consequently she didn't have her spinal curves supported. Her hunched shoulders, her forward-reaching arms, and her flexed head were all evidence of overworked muscles in her upper body. As if all that weren't enough, when JoAnne worked on her computer, her posture became even worse: her monitor had been placed on her desk so that it was to the right of the paperwork, which meant that in order to look at the monitor, Joanne had to turn her head so far to one side that her chin was almost in line with her shoulder.

The Solution:

JoAnne's go-for-broke attitude toward life was great, but it wasn't so great when it was the ergonomic commandments that were being broken – and not just one of them, either. She was breaking so many commandment that it would have taken Moses half an hour to sweep up the pieces! And, of course, she was paying the price.

The cause of the pain in JoAnne's shoulders and neck was as obvious to me as it probably is to you, now that you understand the first five commandments. Still, I had to start at the beginning of the commandments before I could permanently alter her experience of pain. To address her most concerning issue (the pain in her neck and shoulders), I had to systematically fix her poor posture, which would eventually include fixing the major problem caused by her poor head posture while working.

In other words, we had to work one commandment at a time, starting with Commandment #1 – *Secure the Spine*. This didn't make sense to JoAnne, who was concerned about the new pain she had in her neck and shoulders, not the longstanding discomfort in her lower back, but she humoured me and complied with the procedure.

In order to secure the spine, I had to fit JoAnne's chair to her height and lumbar curves. The chair she was using couldn't be adjusted to support her low back curvature, so it was time for her company credit card to spring into action. Even though cost wasn't an issue, we still had to trial a number of different chairs before we found one that could be adjusted specifically to her body size.

The chair height was then raised to align JoAnne's forearms at an angle of 90 degrees to her most frequently used tool, the keyboard. When the seat pan was at the correct height, we found that her feet dangled – things just never seem to run smoothly, do they? But at least that was easy to deal with: a foot rest was provided to support her feet and to further align her thigh/pelvis angles (see Commandment #2 – *Beware the Chair*).

JoAnne's chair was then positioned closer to her keyboard so that her arms were beside her trunk when working (thus making it easy for her shoulders to stop hunching), and after that, the keyboard was repositioned to be a forearm's length away. She was now in compliance with Commandment #3 – *Align the Arms*.

Next we dealt with Commandment #4 – *Watch the Wrist*. To do this, we got rid of JoAnne's old keyboard and bought her a smaller one (without a numeric pad), so that her mouse could be used at an angle that brought it closer to the keyboard. This would keep her arms beside her trunk, in a neutral position. She had been using gel wrist rests, but they encouraged wrist extension so I had no hesitation in getting rid of them. With these changes, I had JoAnne sit at her work station so that I could confirm her wrists were now aligned with her forearms. So far, so good.

Now I turned my attention to her monitor. If Commandment #5 – *Check the Chin* is still fresh in your mind, you'll know that I wanted to have the monitor positioned so that the tool bar on the screen was at the same height as JoAnne's eyebrows. It wasn't, but it only took a moment to raise the screen so it was at the correct height. This would keep her chin parallel to the floor and above her sternal notch.

JoAnn often used the telephone for up to 90 minutes at a time, so naturally her telephone posture was important too. She's right-handed, so we moved the phone so that it was on the left side of the computer, and JoAnne was instructed to answer the phone with her left hand, leaving her right hand free for writing notes when she was taking short telephone calls. This position would also keep her chin parallel to the floor and, I hoped, break her habit of side-flexing her neck in order to hold the telephone between ear and shoulder. JoAnne was also instructed, politely but firmly, to use a headset whenever she was on the phone for a long period of time. She didn't have a headset but she did, of course, have a company credit card, so I made sure that a headset had been purchased before I left the office. Unfortunately no one seems to manufacture a glamorous headset, but from what I saw of JoAnne, I'm sure she soon found a way to make hers look like a fashion accessory. (She could probably have done that by sheer force of personality.) We also ordered a stylish little 3-minute egg timer for her desk, and she promised faithfully to turn it over at the start of every phone call and to put on her headset as soon as the golden sand had all trickled from the top glass bulb to the bottom one. A bit of a gimmick, perhaps, but these things can all act as reminders when we're trying to develop new habits.

Sixth Commandment of Ergonomics
Centre the Nose:

Considering the pain she was having in her neck and upper back, it was important in JoAnne's case to make sure that the monitor and her hard copy were both positioned so that her nose was naturally central to them. Remember, she used the hard copy and the monitor with equal frequency. Looking down at the hard copy on a desk top made her neck flex forward, causing forward compression on the discs in her neck (please see Chapter 5 for an explanation of discs). In addition, because her head was fighting to remain upright against gravity, there was static muscle activity in the muscles of her neck, shoulders and back. So you can see the potential for problems there. And when she was looking at the monitor, JoAnne had to twist her head so far that her chin was almost directly over her shoulder, which caused static muscle activity in different muscle groups as well as torque forces to the discs in her neck. Again, not an ideal situation.

Once we'd noticed JoAnne's nose (and noticed that it wasn't centred to either of her frequent job tasks when she sat at her work station), we had to solve the problem of ensuring that her nose was centred over the monitor, over the hard copy, *and* over the keyboard tray – and what's more, we had to do it stylishly. Did I mention that she didn't want her monitor centred on her desk because she liked to have meetings while sitting at the desk and she thought the monitor was an ugly lump that got in the way? It wasn't that JoAnne was deliberately being difficult, but she was a woman who placed a high value on esthetics. She accepted that she needed to change the position of her monitor, but she didn't want to give it a prime location in the centre of her desk because although she recognized the monitor's usefulness, in her eyes it was primarily a large, unattractive object that didn't complement her surroundings or her working style. How could I make sure that JoAnne's nose was in the correct position and yet still manage to please her? Well, here are the rules for Commandment #6 – *Centre the Nose*, and here's what I did to ensure that JoAnne was working in a correct posture that eliminated her pain.

How do you centre the nose?

Your nose is an important anatomic landmark that can be used to make sure your head position and wrist position are aligned correctly with each other. Follow these steps and you'll be able to notice the position of your own nose and set yourself up to centre it.

Step 1: Monitor: While you're sitting securely in your chair with your keyboard at a 90-degree angle to your elbows, you need to move your monitor so that it's in front of your face. Now look straight at your monitor – pretend it's a mirror. When you look at your face in this "mirror", *notice the nose*. Is it in the middle of your monitor screen? If not, change the height of your monitor, or in other words, *Centre the Nose*. Once your nose is centred, this will automatically place your eyebrows at the height of the tool bar, and your chin will be parallel to the floor (that's Commandment # 5 – *Check the Chin*).

If you have a very pronounced dislike for keeping the monitor in the middle of the desk at all times, I suggest you look into purchasing a movable monitor arm, a clever device that will allow you to swing the monitor away from the middle of the desk whenever you need to utilize that space. JoAnne was happy with this suggestion and it worked well for her, allowing her to hold meetings at an uncluttered desk. And she promised me faithfully that she would always put the monitor back in the correct position afterwards!

How far away should the monitor be?

The monitor should be at a distance that shouldn't cause eyestrain. If it's too close, the muscles around the eyes work hard to accommodate and converge on the images. If it's too far away, the images and characters on the monitor may be difficult to see. Typically, positioning the monitor at arm's length from your seated position (40 to 70 centimeters, or 15 to 27 inches) provides visual comfort for the majority of people. If this distance is too far for you to see images clearly, it's better to increase the font size than to force a shorter viewing distance.

Some people (graphic artists or game designers, for instance) use two computer monitors when working. If you'd like to see in more detail the types of solutions recommended for this set-up, please refer to my web site (www.ergocommandments.ca). For the moment, I'll just point out that if your desk holds two computer monitors that are both used with equal frequency, *centre the nose:* the monitors should be positioned side by side, as close together as possible, and your nose should be centre to the spot where the two monitors meet.

Step 2: Copy Holder: If you spend as much time viewing hard copy as you do viewing the monitor, the hard copy should be placed on a device that doesn't just elevate it but can also position it so the nose is centred over the document in question. I prefer to position the copy directly under the computer monitor so that the head has to flex only minimally and the eyes can look down without strain. I find that an inclined surface works the best.

Step 3: Keyboard: Is keying your most frequent task? When you glance down at the keyboard, *centre your nose* over the letters G and H. The G and H keys should also align with the centre point of your monitor. Failing to properly align the keyboard with other devices is a very common mistake. If your nose is over the G and H on the keyboard, not only does your head benefit but your wrists remain closer to their anatomically neutral position.

Step 4: Phone: A wireless headset is recommended if you have frequent telephone calls, long telephone calls, or frequent long telephone calls ("I've told you, honey, don't call me at the office!"). Any headset should be trialed before purchase, and on-site instructions/training should be provided. Most of the difficulty with a headset is related to its weight (too heavy) or its fit (too big for the ear canal). And remember, a headset is only helpful *if you actually use it*! So consider buying a 3-minute egg timer to remind yourself that it's time to put that headset on.

Regardless of whether or not you use a headset, your telephone should be positioned on the side of your desk opposite to your writing hand. (In other words, if you're right-handed, the phone should be on the left-hand side of your desk.) This way, you can write with one hand while holding the phone in the other, and you won't need to bend your neck to keep the phone in position. I suggest that you use a notebook or some other form of bound paper rather than loose pages, so that you don't need a third hand to hold the paper in place while you write.

What happened to JoAnne?

JoAnne's situation was a challenge in terms of achieving commandment #6 – *Centre the Nose*. I'm happy to report, however, that we managed it in the end. Here's how we did it.

The height of JoAnne's monitor was raised so that if it had been a mirror, her nose would have been at the centre of the reflective surface. Raising the monitor ensured that the tool bar on the screen was at eyebrow height. As you'll recall, JoAnne wasn't happy about this commandment because she conducted meetings at her desk and didn't want the computer to interfere with seeing the person she was meeting with. She described the monitor as ugly, and I can see her point.

To allow JoAnne to work in a correct posture while still satisfying her esthetic requirements, we attached her monitor to a moveable arm, and this device allowed her to swing the monitor away from the middle of the desk when she was in a meeting.

Since JoAnne used hard copy as much as she used the monitor, we had to centre her nose to the hard copy as well as to the monitor. We did this by means of a copy holder – but of course, for JoAnne it couldn't be just any old copy holder. It didn't necessarily have to look like a fashion accessory (although I'm sure she'd have preferred one with a designer label), but it did have to be wide enough to hold the type of files she used, small enough to be placed in the area directly under the monitor, and portable enough to be easily removed from her desk when she was conducting meetings at her desk. It also had to elevate the hard copy enough so that her chin was parallel to the floor when viewing the hard copy. In other words, this was a copy holder that would prevent cervical flexion/rotation and ensure a correct head position when working. Fortunately we were able to find one that met all these criteria, and with all seven of the Commandments implemented, JoAnne is now working in comfort as well as in style.

Summary:

Many computer users get used to ongoing discomfort and tend to ignore it until either discomfort turns to pain in the affected body part or more body parts start to become uncomfortable. Ordinary movement performed too many times, ordinary postures held for long periods, or extreme postures held for short periods can all result in complaints of discomfort.

If discomfort at the work station becomes a concern, please use my system of commandments to ensure you're working in a posture that's anatomically correct, and please also remember to work through the commandments in order, because each one builds on the next. *Centre the Nose* is Commandment #6, but it should be preceded by the first five commandments if you really want to achieve long-term benefit. The spine and the arms are important anatomical landmarks to consider when ensuring your posture is correct, and the previous chapters cover those areas.

Your nose is an important anatomical landmark too. To satisfy the sixth commandment, the nose should align with the centre of your monitor and be lined up to bisect the G and H keys on your keyboard. These adjustments will reinforce the other commandments. For example, placing your nose above the G and H keys will prevent your wrists from moving out of the correct anatomical position, and making sure your nose is central to the monitor will put your eyebrows at toolbar height, which will put you at the correct height to maintain the correct shape of the vertebrae in your neck (cervical curve). Remember that the height of the monitor may vary with the use of glasses, especially progressive lens (please see Commandment #5 – *Check the Chin*).

In these chapters, I've described some of the many ways in which the commandments can be achieved. The equipment you purchase can vary in price depending on your budget (the least expensive item may work as well for you as the most expensive one would have done) and – who knows? – you may even invent a device that the ergonomic world has been waiting for.

Chapter Seven

Commandment Seven

Take a Break

Case History:

The Problem:

I hadn't worked with anyone who had Mary's problem.

For the last five years, she had worked as a paralegal for a large law firm. The poor girl couldn't describe her symptoms to me without crying. Despite taking an alarming number of pain pills, her buttock and thigh symptoms were wreaking havoc with her life. Her pain meant that she couldn't walk normally – she looked stiff as a board when walking, and she moved so slowly and painfully that watching her made my own body ache. She couldn't stand up or sit down without using her arms to either push herself out of the chair or ease herself down into a sitting position. She was only 35 years old. And when she had finally lowered herself onto a chair, her pain was so bad that she couldn't sit there for long anyway. No wonder she kept breaking down and crying.

Mary had been attending physiotherapy treatments in the hope of getting some relief, and she understood from the physiotherapist that her pain resulted from the piriformis muscles located deep in her buttocks. Knowing the source of the pain, however, did nothing to alleviate it. Mary told me that although her buttock pain had developed slowly, it had been unbearable for the last two weeks. She broke down in tears at least a dozen times during the hour-long assessment, especially when describing her inability to work at her former level of productivity. She just couldn't crank out the work the way she used to. If she sat for too long, her whole body felt stiff, and the aching in her legs and spine intensified. She'd had to give up walking to work, and she'd even had to give up walking her dog, an activity that had always helped her to slow down and smell the flowers. The pain drained her of all energy, leaving her exhausted, but its intensity was such that she couldn't sleep. And on top of all of this, because she felt her productivity was low, she wanted to work longer hours to catch up, so she didn't feel she had time to go to the doctor or to continue with physiotherapy or even to take any breaks during the day. Mary was a dedicated employee.

At the beginning of my ergonomic assessment of Mary, I felt stumped. What could I offer her in terms of the seven commandments that would help buttock pain? However, her case turned out to prove to me once again that if you systematically go through each commandment, you *will* improve. You might say (tongue in cheek) that the fact that I was able to help Mary renewed my faith in the commandments. In fact, it was Mary's case that spurred me on to make my commandments public.

Remember, with the Seven Commandments, we always start with a review of the most frequent tasks performed. In Mary's case, her most frequent tasks were evenly split between inputting information into the computer and reading information from the stacks of paperwork that were given to her. She did both these jobs from a seated position, working long hours and never taking breaks – not even a lunch break. Lunch for Mary was just something else that you did at your work station. She had decided some time ago that walking to and from work (30 minutes each way) and walking her dog (20 minutes morning and evening) was all the exercise she needed. What Mary really needed was to build into her work day the seventh commandment, *Take a Break*.

The Solution:

Here's what we did. After we reviewed the first six commandments and identified that Mary needed to take more breaks, we decided to reorganize her work behavior so as to purposefully alternate sitting with standing postures, a change that (in theory) would decrease her pain since these stand-up breaks would counteract the forces through her spine when sitting and the static muscle contraction in her buttock muscles. Since Mary read legal documents for segments totaling half the day, I asked her to always read these documents while standing. As with most people who are faced with the introduction of a change in their work behavior, Mary was somewhat reluctant to try it. She did let me change her work station, though, rearranging it so that all the materials that she had to read were kept on a surface which was at a height that forced her to stand up to access them. It was a relatively modest change, and with gentle encouragement, Mary made a commitment to try it for a month.

When I saw her a month later, I was delighted to observe that Mary was moving much better. She had incorporated the standup breaks into her routine, and now they were a matter of habit. She was still taking pain medication and still going to physiotherapy, but she told me with a smile that her pain had decreased, and I assured her that she was heading in the right direction. Since the pain had taken a long time to build up, I reminded her, the recovery would also take a long time. But it would be worth it.

Seventh Commandment of Ergonomics
Take a Break:

As we've seen, the seventh commandment is *Take a Break*. And as you can imagine, some employers aren't too keen on the sound of this commandment. Some workers worry about it too, especially if they're paid on their output. Taking a break, however, doesn't necessarily mean decreasing productivity. In fact, there are many studies that prove productivity at work actually *increases* after taking a break, and I'll review some of these studies below. Taking a break doesn't necessarily mean stopping work altogether (sorry if I've disappointed you) but rather alternating the muscle groups used. There are many ways to take a break without stopping work: for instance, there are *micro-breaks* where you pause for a few seconds, there are *stretch* breaks where (surprise, surprise) you perform a stretch, and there are *postural* breaks where you change from standing to sitting or vice versa. You can also change postures by incorporating walking into your work day: you can make a habit of walking to the printer after each job instead of waiting for the jobs to accumulate, for example.

If you input data for more than four hours at a time, you *must* get up from a seated posture *at least* once an hour. It's really not that hard to program breaks into your day. Stand every time your telephone rings; walk to the printer to collect a single document; get a glass of water to keep hydrated; perform stretches at the end of each job you complete; persuade your boss to let you take your dog or cat to work. Point out that bending down to pet your furry friend will not only relieve your muscle strain but also lower your blood pressure while raising the level of endorphins in your system, thus making you a much fitter employee. (Hey, it's worth a try.) Taking a break is all about resting the muscles that you use the most, simply by changing which muscles you're using. In Mary's case, it meant routinely performing an activity that was the opposite of sitting. Mary would confirm that taking a break allows the muscles to become energized again and actually boosts productivity. We'll review the types of breaks you can take (and the reasons you need to take them) below. Don't break yet, LOL!

MSI with too much movement and MSI with too little movement:

Many of the people I see for ergonomic assessments don't take regular breaks. They drink their coffee at their desk, skip lunch, and seldom go home on time at the end of the work day. When I perform worksite visits and recommend that clients take a break from their work more regularly, they invariably say that they don't have time because they have too much work to do. Mary said the same thing, until she learned that not taking breaks made her less productive rather than more.

In many of the interviews I conduct, the history I hear is the same, and by now you know the general outline of the story: the body invariably gave the computer user many clues before the pain became incapacitating. The clues were easy to ignore, so that's just what happened: they were ignored. After a while, one particular body part grew more noticeable at the end of a work day. Tired of being ignored, the body was nagging. And when your body nags like that, you need to pay attention. You shouldn't be more aware of any particular body part at the end of the day, because that's a story with only one ending: this nagging discomfort will amplify and turn into pain.

You know from all the preceding chapters that computer-related musculoskeletal injuries (MSIs) result from ordinary, innocent little movements that are repeated over and over again, every working day, for years. MSI is a phenomenon that occurs silently as we gain more computer experience – and, of course, as we age. The longer you use the computer, the more dangerous that computer becomes, as the effects of all the ordinary little movements sneak up on you. The risk of having to deal with an MSI is one that exponentially increases with age. Remember, the silent epidemic of MSI occurred after 10 years of computer use!

Most people, if they think about computer-related injuries at all, assume they only occur in the fingers, hands, and wrists. It's an understandable assumption because those are the body parts that are most visibly being used for repetitive movement via keyboarding or mousing. Other body parts, however, are affected by what they're *not* doing while working on that computer. Think about Mary's situation as described above. For hours on end, every working day, she sat with her back, shoulders and head held in one position while her hands did all the work. The result? MSI *not* in the fingers, hands, or wrists, where you would expect it, but in the large muscle groups that supported her posture for so long. I'm the first to admit that Mary's buttock pain was an unusual MSI: pain in the back muscles or shoulders is a far more common symptom. But Mary's pain proves that pain can be caused by *some* ordinary movements being performed too *many* times and *other* ordinary movements being performed too *few* times, without giving the poor old muscles a break. If you add poor posture into the mix, plus the requirement for the muscles to exert force (remember: the more forces, the greater the danger), combined with a lack of rest for those working muscles, you have a great recipe for MSI. You might say that Mary tossed those ingredients into her body's slow cooker a long time ago, and eventually she had to deal with the results. What ingredients have you been putting into *your* body's slow cooker?

These types of MSI injuries didn't arise when we were all using typewriters, and we discussed the reasons for this a little earlier in the book. Mostly it was because of the forced micro-breaks the typist took (quite unintentionally) while changing paper, correcting mistakes, etc. These actions were trivial, but they did cause small changes in the typist's posture, and those small changes in posture gave the body a chance for physiological recovery.

Anatomy Lesson –

The Importance of Breaks:

Our bodies are made to move. Muscles move our bodies, and muscles work best when they're moving our joints dynamically. And although it sounds counterintuitive, it's movement that provides the muscles with a chance to recuperate.

Here's how that works. Dynamic movements are characterized by a rhythmic alternation of muscle contraction and extension, tension and relaxation. Walking is a classic example. Contraction of the muscle results in compression, which squeezes blood out of the muscle, and the subsequent relaxation releases a fresh flow of blood into the muscle. In effect, the muscle is acting as a pump in the blood system. The muscle is flushed with incoming blood, which lets it retain its energy; at the same time, waste products are removed by the outgoing blood. This explains why you feel so good after you finish a walk. Your muscles are working, and energy is being funneled in as fast as it is being used. You are, quite literally, "pumped".

Now let's take a look at walking versus working. How much dynamic muscle contraction is going on when you're working on your computer? If we look at your trunk, arms or neck, we can't see much movement happening, so if your answer to the preceding question was "Not a lot," you'd be right. But as you know, that doesn't mean your muscles are taking a break when you do desk work – far from it. Even though there's virtually no movement of your joints, your muscles are working – and working fairly hard, I might add – to hold your body upright against the effects of gravity. In this state of *static muscle activity*, the muscles stay in a prolonged state of contraction or heightened tension. And a prolonged state of heightened physical tension is no better for our muscles than a prolonged state of heightened mental tension is for our minds.

In static muscle activity, the blood vessels are compressed by the muscle tissue so that blood no longer flows through in volume, which means that the muscle isn't receiving as many nutrients from the blood, nor is it able to eliminate as many waste products. You could say that the muscle is constipated. When they're in that state, muscles become "naggy" – that is, they're trying to attract your attention, and with good reason: they want to be re-energized, they want to be "pumped", and that's not going to happen if you don't move.

It's one thing if static muscle contraction occurs when the joints are stacked nicely on top of each other, as they are in the spine, but it's more complicated if the static contraction involves the muscles having to support a weighted object against the downward force of gravity: for example, your shoulder muscles having to support the weight of your outstretched arm. Because the arm acts as a lever, the shoulder muscles must work harder to support its weight, and the effects of fatigue set in more quickly. Remember, every time you move out of anatomical alignment, static muscle activity occurs. Mousing is a good example. Mousing doesn't take much energy unless you hold your arm away from your trunk and use a straight elbow when you operate the mouse. In that position, when your shoulder is out of its resting position and the arm is not moving, static muscle contraction occurs in your shoulder, and you use an exorbitant amount of energy to fight gravity as a result. The blood supply to the shoulder muscles is compromised due to *static muscle activity.* And you know how the story goes from there: first, a little shoulder discomfort when you use the mouse; next, your shoulder starting to nag you by the end of the day. And if you don't give those muscles a break, sooner or later that "naggy" feeling is going to become pain. To work optimally, your muscles must be supplied with energy, and you know what that means: gotta get that blood flowing through!

Many people have no idea how hard their muscles are having to work in static muscle activity (did you know that static muscle contraction increases your heartbeat to a higher rate than dynamic muscle contractions do?), and so when they start to feel tired, they compensate in ways that use even *more* energy and create even *more* fatigue. For instance, tired muscles can lead to slouching, which in turn can lead to worse posture. Poor posture uses more energy and creates more fatigue. It becomes a chronic cycle. Rest breaks, on the other hand, allow the body to recover and the energy to flow back to the muscles, so that we feel less tired. And when I say "rest break", I'm not talking about taking a siesta, or even a catnap. "A change is as good as a rest" should be a mantra for all computer users.

The "break" principle also applies to dynamic movements. While they're better for your body than static movements, performing too many dynamic movements for too long has its own inherent problems, because when a part of the body (the hand or wrist, let's say) is used repetitively to the point of overuse, soft tissue begins to break down on a cellular level. At an internal level – a level we're not even consciously aware of – our body needs to regenerate our cells. During a repetitive task, pauses enable the cells to regenerate; not taking pauses lets them deteriorate. The choice is yours.

There's a fine line between too much movement and not enough movement, but it's *always* true that maintaining a good posture and taking rest breaks is sensible preventative medicine. In terms of muscle energy, your goal is to make sure that input and output match, but the good news is that this can be accomplished in mere seconds! You just need to build in *micro-breaks*.

What constitutes a break? What types of break are there?

Most employees working an eight-hour shift are entitled to two 15-minute breaks and one 30-minute meal period, a standard practice that breaks up the work shift in order to give employees a chance to rest and become refreshed. Providing additional, shorter rest breaks each hour has been shown to further reduce the risk of discomfort, fatigue, and injury, but I must admit that I don't know any employers who actually implement this (although I probably know a few whose employees cheerfully implement it on their behalf).

How often should breaks be taken? Well, numerous studies have been conducted to determine not just how frequently they should be taken but what actually constitutes an optimal break, both for our health and for productive work. The results may surprise you.

Probably the most important of these studies was conducted in 1997 by Henning *et al.*[xi] In this study, 92 computer users were observed while they performed typing tasks. Their performance was measured in three different ways: when they took their traditional breaks, when they were given three 30-second micro-breaks, and when the micro breaks were coupled with brief stretching exercises.

Results showed that not only did these micro-breaks help minimize postural injury risks, but *when micro-breaks were combined with stretching, productivity actually increased by 14.9%*. These results indicate that (a) the body performs better when it has the opportunity to re-energize via micro-breaks and (b) the re-energizing is especially effective when micro-breaks are coupled with appropriate stretches.

In a more recent study of data-entry operators, a comparison was made between a standard rest break schedule and one that had a 5-minute rest break during each hour. The hourly rest break schedule resulted in a reduction in eyestrain and discomfort to the forearm, wrist, and hand, *without a reduction in data-entry performance.* [xii] And if you think it's impressive that the group that took more breaks was able to do the same amount of work, consider this: the greatest difference between the two groups was in *the last hour of work.*

What's particularly interesting is that, in the last hour of work, not only did the group that did *not* take the extra breaks demonstrate the most fatigue, they also had the greatest decrease in productivity. So taking extra breaks can lead to a win-win situation: the employees win because they feel less tired, and the employer wins because productivity stays high throughout the day. Be aware, however, that fatigue has a cumulative effect, so you can't ward off fatigue by saving up all your breaks until the last part of the day – that kind of shortcut doesn't boost your productivity. The breaks have to be taken *throughout* the day in order for your body to benefit. If you skip your breaks during the day, you'll end up working harder *and* becoming more fatigued toward the end of the day.

When you're tired, you're more likely to injure yourself, as I'm sure you know from personal experience. The effects of poor posture, repetitive movements, and static movements can catch up with you much more quickly when your muscles are fatigued. This may not only predispose you to an MSI at work but may result in you being unable to enjoy your activities after work, thus adding mental stress to your physical stress.

What are the different ways you can take a rest break? A *micro-break* is the quickest form of break: you just stop whatever you're doing, count to 30, and start again. Micro-breaks last 30 to 60 seconds and are recommended every 10 minutes if you're doing a highly repetitive task.

Then there's the *mini-break*, which lasts three to five minutes and which, if performed every 30 to 60 minutes, gives your body a rest, reduces discomfort, and improves performance. Rather than requiring you to stop work altogether, mini-breaks can consist of alternating your work activities and postures throughout the day. You can take a mini-break simply by walking to the printer, getting a glass of water, or standing up to answer the phone. Some people find it helpful to actually program mini-breaks into their day rather than performing them as the occasion arises. Alternating your tasks may seem inefficient, and it will certainly feel strange at first, but the use of different muscle groups really will increase energy and productivity. (If you don't believe me, look up for yourself the studies that I cited earlier.) Remember, Mary's pain was relieved by something as simple as training herself to stand up whenever she read something, thus automatically providing her muscles with a much-needed break from long periods of sitting.

There's also the *stretch break*, which is just what it sounds like: you just stretch during your work tasks. You might not know it, but there are many stretch-prompting programs that can be downloaded onto your computer free of charge and will not only remind you to stretch but will show you *how* to stretch appropriately. You're not aiming for a workout: gentle stretching will do a fine job of providing muscle relief and a time for recovery. Stretches don't just increase your flexibility, they also promote the flow of blood, which in turn promotes the flow of oxygen and thus the flow of energy to the muscles. Just standing up to stretch after sitting for long periods of time has recuperative value because it improves circulation, allows the exchange of nutrients between the spinal discs and surrounding tissue, and compensates for having spent time in a static posture.

Summary:

I've now reviewed the causes of MSI and the effects of too many movements and too few movements. In other chapters of this book, we spent time examining the importance of correct anatomical posture in order to prevent MSI, but this is the first time we've focused on the importance of rest and how a rest can be obtained simply by changing your body position or alternating your body actions, i.e., taking a break. That's the seventh commandment of ergonomics – *Take a Break*. Too much of a good thing is no longer good, right? Taking a break will increase your productivity and ultimately keep you healthy. Build micro-breaks into your daily routine. Take those mini-breaks and stretch breaks. Stand every time the telephone rings. Walk to the printer. Get a glass of water. Download a free stretching program and perform the exercises regularly to stretch commonly used muscles.

I'm not telling you this just to scare you, but I do want you to think – and think seriously – about taking breaks and allowing your body to move. Don't just think about it: *do it*! Your body deserves a break, and you won't slow down in your work: you'll be more productive. So you have nothing to lose and everything to gain by incorporating breaks into your daily office routine.

CHAPTER EIGHT

Using the Seven Commandments of Ergonomics

The Problem:

Computer-related injuries are a global concern spanning all age groups. Research shows that work-related soft tissue injuries are the most frequent cause for losing time off work; they're also the largest source of lost-time worker compensation costs in Canada. If you project this information to the rest of the world and consider that at least 50% of the world's population works in some form of office, you realize that computer-related pain is already disrupting many livelihoods. If you further project this information to the reality that computer use is advancing with lightning speed through all age groups and socio-economic classes, it's easy to foresee computer-related injury growing to pandemic proportions.

The Solution:

I formulated the Seven Commandments of Ergonomics over a period of 25 years, after performing many, many ergonomic assessments dealing with many, many computer-related problems. I've assessed hundreds of clients in hundreds of offices, and the overwhelming majority of the complaints I've dealt with have originated with incorrect posture – how the person was sitting and where their most frequently used equipment was situated. My Seven Commandments of Ergonomics therefore always begin by looking at the person's posture when they're sitting. After the seated posture is changed so that anatomical perfection is achieved, my next job is to identify the most repetitive task performed in the job. I then look at the equipment used to carry out the most repetitive task, and I reposition or change the equipment to ensure that mid range of motion is achieved in all joints if anatomical perfection cannot be maintained.

My system involves a total of seven crucial steps – the Seven Commandments of Ergonomics. These seven steps aren't just rules: they're more important than that, which is why I called them commandments. I have used these commandments more often in the last couple of years, and I suspect this is due to the proliferation of computers, the increasing age of the workforce, and the cumulative effects of incorrect computer use. There is an overwhelming amount of literature about ergonomics that one can research, but I've done the research for you and grouped the information into a system you can use that involves seven sequential commandments. I have worked with these commandments for a long time, and now I'm sharing them with you. These commandments are all about keeping you working in a correct anatomical posture, starting with how you sit on your chair. Considering the breadth of possible computer-related injuries, if even 1% of the computer-using population were to use these commandments and work with better posture, literally millions of people would receive benefit. My research and experience will have benefitted more people than I can work with single-handed! Please use these Seven Commandments of Ergonomics, and we could work together to **ESC Computer Pain.**

Here is a checklist with at-a-glance instructions that you can use to adjust your own work station. Bear in mind that if you don't change your work station in the order given, starting with the first commandment and working your way down the list, you'll find yourself rearranging your workspace a multiple number of times - far more than seven! – and I can say that with confidence because believe me, I've been there and done that, so you might as well profit from my mistakes.

Please don't change anything about your work station until you perform a full assessment. Work through the instructions listed under each commandment. Before you change anything, you need to identify all the areas where ergonomic intervention is necessary – *assess first*. Then, and only then, do you change anything! When you do start making changes (after you've gone through the checklist for each commandment and identified where changes need to be made), always start with Commandment #1 and correct all the deficit areas under each commandment in turn. In some instances, you may find that your posture changes to such an extent that the deficit areas you had previously identified have self-corrected. Bonus!!

The goals of each commandment are summarized for you, followed by the details on how to comply. This isn't a test, so please feel free to re-read any of the relevant chapters if you have questions.

The Seven Commandments of Ergonomics:

1. **Secure the Spine**: How to ensure anatomically correct head, back and lower extremity posture when seated.

2. **Beware the Chair**: How to fit you and your chair to your computer work station.

3. **Align the Arms**: How to position your shoulders in a rest position and your elbows in mid range of motion while performing your most frequent tasks.

4. **Watch the Wrist**: What to look for to make sure your wrist is in optimal position so that you avoid computer-related injury.

5. **Check the Chin**: How to correctly position your head in relation to your computer screen, your keyboard, and your work space, using your chin as a landmark.

6. **Centre the Nose**: How to position your head correctly in relation to the keyboard and monitor, using your nose as a reference.

7. **Take a Break**: What is a break and how often should you take one?

The Seven Commandments of Ergonomics Checklist and Instructions for Use:

Step 1: – Know Where To Start:

Knowing where to start is often the hardest part! Identify your most repetitive task and begin your ergonomic assessment with that task in mind. Assess first; that means you read all the steps under each commandment and fill in the boxes. You must fully understand what's wrong before you implement the changes required to put it right.

Step 2: – The Checklist:

Fill out the checklist below, using an X to identify areas that need attention.

Commandment #1: Secure the Spine.

Stand while you answer the first question below, and then sit down in your chair to answer the remaining questions, inserting ☑ if your work station complies and ☒ if the area needs attention.

☐ Is the bottom of your kneecap at the same height as the seat pan of your chair?

☐ Is there room for a fist between your calf and the edge of your chair when seated?

☐ Is the lumbar support on the chair adjusted correctly? Is your low back curve filled?

☐ Is your ear aligned directly over your shoulder?

☐ Is your shoulder aligned directly above your hip?

Commandment #2: **Beware the Chair.**

Now pull your chair in front of your work surface and answer these questions.

☐ Can your chair be rolled easily to your work surface?

☐ Keep your elbows tucked beside your trunk and bend your elbows to 90 degrees. Is your keyboard positioned at your fingertips?

☐ Keep your elbows tucked beside your trunk and bend your elbows to 90 degrees. Is your mouse positioned at your fingertips?

☐ Do the arm rests of your chair allow you to work with your elbows beside your trunk?

☐ Do the arm rests of your chair rest directly below your 90-degree elbow and keep your arms close to your trunk?

☐ Do your arm rests allow your chair to be pulled forearm's distance away from your desk?

☐ Are your feet flat on the floor?

☐ If you use a foot rest, does it support both feet?

☐ If you use a foot rest, is it stable?

☐ Is the monitor directly over the keyboard?

☐ Are the items that you use frequently (> 8 x hour) at forearm's distance?

☐ Are the items that you use on an occasional basis at arm's reach?

Commandment #3: **Align the Arms.**

Briefly perform your most frequent task, and then answer these questions.

☐ Is your arm beside and close to your trunk when you're keyboarding?

☐ Is your arm beside and close to your trunk when you're mousing?

☐ Is your elbow at 90 degrees when you're keyboarding?

☐ Is your elbow at 90 degrees when you're mousing?

☐ When you're using the arm rests, are your forearms horizontal and your shoulders relaxed?

Commandment #4: **Watch the Wrist.**

Briefly perform your most frequent task once again, and then answer these questions.

☐ Is your wrist in neutral position (in other words, your thumb in line with your forearm) when you're typing?

☐ Is it in neutral position when you're mousing?

☐ Is your middle knuckle aligned central to your forearm when typing and mousing?

☐ Is there an absence of contact pressure?

☐ Does the angle of your keyboard allow you to maintain your wrist in a neutral position?

Commandment #5: **Check the Chin.**

Check the relationship between the monitor and your head, using the chin for a reference point.

☐ Is your monitor positioned in front of you so that if the monitor was a mirror, your nose would be in the centre of it?

☐ Is the on-screen toolbar at the same height as your eyebrows?

☐ Is your chin positioned over your sternal notch?

☐ Is your chin parallel to the floor?

☐ Is your monitor at arm's reach (that is, at a distance of 15 to 27 inches from you)?

☐ Is your monitor free of glare?

☐ Is your hard copy positioned on either side of the monitor or else directly below the monitor?

☐ Do your glasses allow you to maintain a chin position that's parallel to the floor?

Commandment #6: **Centre the Nose**.

Check the relationship of your head in relation to your monitor and keyboard.

☐ Is your nose in the centre of your computer screen?

☐ Is your nose centred over the letters G and H on your keyboard?

Commandment #7: Take a Break.

Are you providing a chance for your body to recover?

- ☐ If you input data for more than four hours at a time, are you getting up from a seated posture at least once an hour?

- ☐ Are you regularly taking positional changes, micro-breaks and mini-breaks?

- ☐ Are you stretching throughout the day?

- ☐ Are you taking breaks away from your desk for lunch and coffee?

Step 3: – BEGIN INTERVENTION:

Now that you've identified where you need to make ergonomic changes, the next step, naturally enough, is to make those changes. Let's turn all those X's into check marks! As always, start with Commandment #1 and work your way through to Commandment #7. Refer back to the chapters in the easy-to-use "how to" sections. (One word of caution, however. If you buy new equipment as a result of the Seven Commandments of Ergonomics assessment, make sure you can return the equipment if it turns out not to be suitable for you. Many chair dealers, for example, will lend you a chair to trial. Keyboards and mice are often slightly more difficult to return, however, so make sure you have this discussion with the supplier before you purchase.)

After implementing any necessary changes, most people report feeling awkward initially, because they've been working incorrectly for so long that those unnatural positions have come to feel correct. However, other people report immediate comfort. Where are you on that scale?

Step 4: – FOLLOW UP:

Once you've made these changes, stick with them for *at least* three days and preferably a week. If you're not feeling more comfortable at the end of that time, try redoing the assessment – did you find all the ergonomic problems the first time? Did you reposition your equipment properly?

Congratulations! You have now completed your **Seven Commandments of Ergonomics** assessment and intervention.

Summary:

I believe that people want to work; I believe that being a worker is one of the most important roles in a life; and I believe that people should be able to work without pain and discomfort for as many years as they want to. The information I've shared with you will, I firmly believe, help you to **ESC Computer Pain**. Why go on fighting the effects of gravity on repetition, force and posture? Especially when you know that it's a battle you can't win!

These Seven Commandments will default your posture into an anatomically correct one. Implementing them will be of benefit to you in three ways: it will help you to ward off any computer-related pain that may be silently stalking you; it will enable you to reduce any computer-related pain you may already be experiencing; and it will allow you to work smarter so that you can play harder.

Thank you for letting me share my knowledge and experience with you. I wish you the very best in health, pain-free computer use, and a work history as long as you want it to be.

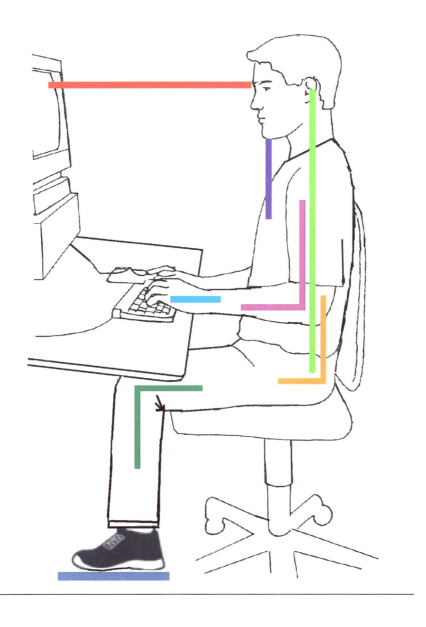

ABOUT THE AUTHOR:

IRENE CHAPPELL is an Occupational Therapist, a Certified Work Capacity Evaluator and an Assistant Clinical Professor at the University of British Columbia. She is the founder of OT CONSULTING/TREATMENT SERVICES LTD.

In 1986, OT CONSULTING/TREATMENT SERVICES LTD. was the first private practice occupational therapy clinic in British Columbia to develop and implement work assessment and treatment programs. Today, the clinic employs 35 specialists who provide services in the assessment, treatment, and prevention of work-related injury. We're proud of pioneering an industry that not only keeps growing but keeps improving the lives of others.

Irene has lectured in return-to-work issues and ergonomics at the School of Rehabilitation Sciences (Occupational Therapy and Physiotherapy Divisions) at the University of British Columbia. She has appeared as a guest speaker at conferences throughout Canada and internationally in Australia, England, and Hong Kong. She is a recognized authority on the evaluation and development of work potential.

Irene has consulted on and designed ergonomic programmes for a variety of industries and businesses, including legal firms, banking and educational institutions, the forestry sector, government municipalities, bakeries and unions.

She has been recognized by the Supreme Court of British Columbia as an expert in return-to-work issues, ergonomics and the costing of future care needs. She has been published in the *Canadian Journal of Occupational Therapy*; *Continuing Legal Education Society of B.C.*; *Rehab Review*; *People Talk*; and various other trade journals. Irene is also a co-author of the book entitled *The Functional Capacity Evaluation: A Clinician's Guide*.

Bibliography:

Balance Systems, Inc. (2006). *Balance Systems, Inc.* Retrieved February 2011, from Advance Research in Rehabilitation Technology: http://www.repetitive-strain.com/cts/ctsindex.html

Canadian Centre for Occupational Health and Safety. (2007, July). *Canadian Centre for Occupational Health and Safety.* Retrieved July 2011, from Sitting on the Job and the Risks of Deep Vein Thrombosis, Health and Safety Report, Volume 5, Issue 4: http://www.ccohs.ca/newsletters/hsreport/issues/2007/04/ezine.html#inthenews

Canadian Centre for Occupational Health and Safety (n.d.). *Canadian Centre for Occupational Health and Safety.* Retrieved January 2011, from Canadian Centre for Occupational Health and Safety Web site: http:/www.ccohs.ca/oshanswsers/ergonomics/office/chair_adjusting.html

Cluett, J. M. (n.d.). *About.Com Orthopedics*. Retrieved August 2011, from Carpal Tunnel Syndrome Treatment, What treatments are available for carpal tunnel syndrome?: http://orthopedics.about.com/cs/carpaltunnel/a/carpaltunnel_3.htm

Cornell University Web (n.d.). *Cornell University Web.* Retrieved March 2011, from CUErgo, Ergonomic Guidelines for aranging a Computer Work Station - 10 steps for users: http://ergo.human.cornell.edu/ergoguide.html

Dababneh, A., S. N. (2001, February). Impact of added rest breaks on the productivity and well being of workers. *Ergonomics 44(2)*, pp. 164-174.

National Institute of Neurological Disorders and Stroke (n.d.). *National Institute of Neurological Disorders and Stroke.* Retrieved February 2011, from National Institute of Neurological Disorders and Stroke: 2011.http://www.ninds.nih.gov/disorders/carpal_tunnel/det ail_carpal_tunnel.htm

State Compensation Insurance Fund (n.d.). *State Compensation Insurance Fund.* Retrieved July 2012, from Additional Rest Breaks Show Reduction in Fatigue and Injury, ErgoMatters, Volume 4, Number 3: http://www.statefundca.com/safety/ErgoMatters/Micro-breaks.asp

State Compensation Insurance Fund (n.d.). *State Compensation Insurance Fund.* Retrieved July 2012, from Micro-breaks, ErgoMatters, Volume 3, Number 4: http://www.statefundca.com/safety/ErgoMatters/Micro-breaks.asp

State Compensation Insurance Fund (n.d.). *State Compensation Insurance Fund.* Retrieved July 2012, from Ergonomic Breaks, Rest Periods and Stretches: http://www.statefundca.com/safety/safetymeeting/SafetyM eetingArticle.aspx?ArticleID=357

Tieldman, Jeff (n.d.). *State Compensation Insurance Fund.* Retrieved July 2012, from New Concepts in Seating: http://www.statefundca.com/safety/SeatingConcepts.asp.

References:

i. Carswell, C.M. (Ed.). Review of human factors and ergonomics (4) *Human Factors and Ergonomics Society.* Adapted from Brand, J.L. (2008) Office Ergonomics; Pertinent research and recent developments (245-282).

ii. Health and Safety Executive (n.d.). *Health and Safety Exexcutive,* Retrieved from Musculoskeletal Disorders (MSDs) in Great Britain (GB): //www.hse.gov.uk/statistics/causdis/musculoskeletal/index. htm.

iii. Buckle, P., & Devereux, J., (1999). Work-related Neck and Upper Limb Musculoskeletal Disorders. *European Agency for Safety and Health at Work.*

iv. Bureau of Labor Statistics (n.d.). *Bureau of Labor Statistics.* Retrieved from Injuries, Illnesses and Fatalities: http:/www.bls.gov/iif/

v. Marcus, M. et al. (2002). A prospective study of computer users: II. Postural risk factors for musculoskeletal disorders. *American Journal of Industrial Medicine, (41):* 236-249.

vi. Gerr et al (2002). A prospective study of computer users: I. Study design and incidence of musculoskeletal symptoms and disorders. *American Journal of Industrial Medicine, (41):* 22-235.

vii. Andersen, J.H., Thomsen, J.F., Overgaard, E., et al. (2003). Computer use and carpal tunnel syndrome: A 1-year follow-up study. *JAMA (289):* 2963-2969.

viii. Andersen, J.H., Thomsen, J.F., Overgaard, E., et al (2003). Computer use and carpal tunnel syndrome: A 1-year follow-up study. *JAMA (289):* 2963-2969.

ix.   Berolo, S., Wells, R.P., & Amick III, B. (2011). Musculoskeletal symptoms among mobile hand-held device users and their relationship to device use: A preliminary study in a Canadian University population. *Applied Ergonomics (42):* 371-378.

x.   Brewer, S., Van Erg, D., Amick, B.C., Irvin, E., Daum, K., Gerr, F., Moore, J.S., Cullen, K., & Rempel, D. (2006). Workplace interventions to prevent musculoskeletal and visual symptoms and disorders among computer users: A systematic review. *J Occupational Rehab (3)* 317- 350.

xi.   Henning, R.A., Callaghan, E.A., Ortega, A.M., Kissel, G.V., Guttman, J.I., & Braun, H.A., (1996). Continuous feedback to promote self-management of rest breaks during computer use. *International Journal of Industrial Ergonomics (18):* 71-82.

Henning, R.A., Jacques, P., Kissel, G.V., Sullivan, A.B. & Alteras-Webb, S. (1997). Frequent short rest breaks from computer work: effects on productivity and well-being at two field sites. *Ergonomics (1)*: 78-91.

xii.   Galinsky, T., Swanson, N., et al (2001). A field study of supplementary rest breaks for data-entry operators. *Ergonomics (5):* 622- 638.

Galinsky, T., Swanson, N., et al. (2007). Supplementary breaks and stretching exercises for data entry operators: a follow-up field study. *American Journal of Industrial Medicine (7):* 519-527.

www.ingramcontent.com/pod-product-compliance
Lightning Source LLC
Chambersburg PA
CBHW041142050326
40689CB00001B/448